DEEP BRAIN STIMULATION

DEEP BRAIN STIMULATION

A New Treatment Shows Promise in the Most Difficult Cases

Jamie Talan

DANA PRESS

New York • Washington, D.C.

THE DANA FOUNDATION
745 Fifth Avenue, Suite 900
New York, New York 10151

DANA PRESS
The Dana Center
900 15th Street, NW
Washington, D.C. 20005

DANA is a federally registered trademark.

ISBN-13: 978-1-932594-37-9

This publication is designed to provide accurate and authoritative information in regard to the subject matter covered. It is sold with the understanding that the publisher is not engaged in rendering professional services. If professional advice or other expert assistance is required, the services of a competent professional person should be sought.

Library of Congress Cataloging-in-Publication Data
    Talan, Jamie.
        Deep brain stimulation / by Jamie Talan.
            p. ; cm.
        Includes bibliographical references and index.
        ISBN 978-1-932594-37-9 (cloth : alk. paper)
        1. Brain stimulation. I. Title.
        [DNLM: 1. Deep Brain Stimulation. 2. Brain Diseases—therapy. 3. Movement Disor-
            ders—therapy. WB 495 T137d 2009]
QP388.T35 2009
612.8'26—dc22
                            2008046916

Text design by William Stilwell
Cover design by Tobias' Outerwear for Books

www.dana.org

Contents

ACKNOWLEDGMENTS

A book about one medical technique is not the usual fare. But telling the story of deep brain stimulation allowed me to step back into history and figure out where and how the use of electrical brain stimulators to fix broken movements and minds began. It is the story of scientists, doctors, and brave patients, and thus everyone who took the time to tell me their story deserves big thanks. That includes many people who didn't make the final cut, including George Doeschner and Margaret Fleming. George Doeschner has Parkinson's, and I happened to be visiting him in the hospital when his deep brain stimulator short-circuited and shut down. The battery device used to turn the machine on was with his wife, who was forty minutes away. He had just undergone surgery for a broken arm, one of the many causalities of living off balance with Parkinson's. He was shaking uncontrollably, and it is an undeniable truth about the nature of this device that it can fail someone at any moment. And Margaret Fleming was an artist with essential tremor who showed me how easy it was to have two holes in your head and a battery device in your chest and go about a creative life.

As I would come to understand, there are many histories—and the material in this book is no different. My journey began over tea with Dr. Ron Alterman, who told me about this maverick surgeon (Irving S. Cooper) who started taking patients into his operating room decades ago to help their crumpled bodies attempt to follow the normal, smooth commands of movement that most of us take for granted. I thank Dr. Alim-Louis Benabid, a gentleman and a surgeon who is called the father of deep brain stimulation. A special thanks to Dr. Jerry Vitek, who served as my informal advisor. There are so many people who helped tell the story of this unusual medical technique—you will meet them all in this book. A special thanks to Sissel Cooper, who shared her husband's books and stories. Thanks to my friends and colleagues Dr. Kevin Tracey and Dr. David Eidelberg, who inspire my passion for the brain by the findings that continue to emerge from their labs. Also, thanks to my professional family at the Feinstein Institute for Medical Research. Thanks to Dana editor Dan Gordon, and a special thanks to Jane Nevins, my editor on this book. I have known Jane and the Dana Foundation for more than twenty years, and I appreciate everything that she has done to educate people about the most interesting, complex, beautiful, and damning organ of the human body. To my family, for their enduring love and constant stimulation of my brain.

In the chapter on obsessive-compulsive disorder, you will meet Mario Della Grotta, a 40-year-old who struggled his entire adult life with endless obsessive-compulsive disorder (OCD) symptoms. He fought so hard against the disease that he signed on as the first person in the U.S. with OCD to undergo experimental deep brain stimulation. It helped enormously. Unfortunately, on January 5, 2009, Mario, a husband and father of two small children, passed away from a short medical illness that had nothing to do with his OCD or the stimulators implanted in his brain. I dedicate this book to Mario—for his courage, his inspiration and his unstoppable quest to live a normal life.

Illustrations

The Basal Ganglia

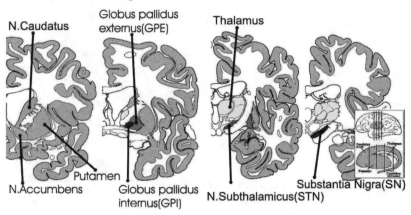

N.Caudatus

Globus pallidus externus(GPE)

Thalamus

Putamen

N.Accumbens

Globus pallidus internus(GPI)

N.Subthalamicus(STN)

Substantia Nigra(SN)

The basal ganglia are important brain structures involved in movement and many diverse physical and mental operations. Scientists are trying these different structures as sites to stimulate with the deep brain stimulator electrodes in treating a wide range of disorders. For example, DBS relieves symptoms for many patients with Parkinson's with the electrodes implanted in the globus pallidus internus.

Brodmann Area 25

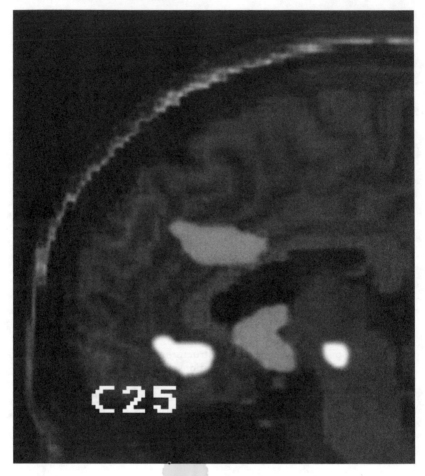

Brodmann area 25 is located in the prefrontal cortex, a brain area involved in higher-level mental operations, and has been implicated in depression. Scientists are investigating area 25 as a target for deep brain stimulation in cases of depression that have not responded to any other treatment. See Chapter 7.

(Courtesy of Helen S. Mayberg, M.D., FRCPC)

Deep brain stimulation

Pacemaker-like devices deliver electrical stimulation to targeted areas in the brain, blocking signals that cause the disabling motor symptoms associated with Parkinson's disease.

1 A surgeon drills two holes in the patient's skull and threads a lead, or insulated wire, with electrodes at the tip to the brain

2 A lead is threaded under the skin from the brain to the upper chest

3 The lead is attached to two pacemaker-like devices called neurostimulators that are surgically implanted in the chest and provide electricity to stimulate the brain

4 An external programmer adjusts the settings of the neurostimulators to ensure the right amount of electricity is delivered to the brain

5 Because the neurostimulators each contain a battery with a limited lifespan, they must be surgically replaced every three to five years

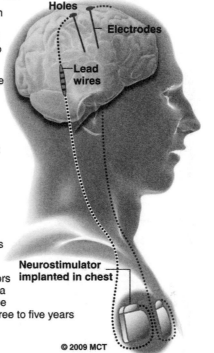

Holes

Electrodes

Lead wires

Neurostimulator implanted in chest

Source: Medtronic Inc., Star Tribune
Graphic: Minneapolis Star Tribune

© 2009 MCT

The first successful applications of deep brain stimulation began with the scientific understanding of the brain in Parkinson's disease and drew on the technical expertise of engineers with the heart-pacemaker manufacturer, Medtronic, Inc.

Prologue

O n March 14, 1997, the U.S. Food and Drug Administration
held a hearing on the use of deep brain stimulation (DBS)
as a treatment for essential tremor and Parkinson's disease. By
that time, excitement about this technology, which could restore
a body to its rightful state of controlled movement, had spread
through brain research laboratories and neurology clinics around
the world. Desperate patients with all kinds of movement disorders had heard about deep brain stimulation, too, and they were
clamoring for access to the treatment.

On this day in March, two American patients, Maurice Long
and George Shafer, were standing before an advisory panel
commissioned by the FDA to study the benefits and risks of deep
brain stimulation. Long and Shafer were among the 83 people
with essential tremor and 113 people with Parkinson's tremor
who had undergone deep brain stimulation in a large clinical trial.
The FDA-approved study was sponsored by Medtronic, the
Minneapolis-based company that supplied the stimulating electrodes for the trial. Founded in 1949 to usher in a new technology
called cardiac pacing, Medtronic had made the first implantable
heart pacemaker. Now the company was in the middle of an

international push on another frontier: the brain seemed to be as receptive to electrical stimulation as the heart.

Maurice Long of Hutchinson, Kansas, traveled to Maryland to testify before the FDA panel. His gait was steady and his hands were at ease as he stood and told the panel, along with dozens of others gathered at the hearing, about the years when he was crippled by essential tremor. It had begun fifteen years earlier, when Long was fifty-seven and worked as a district manager for a financial services company. His hands had started shaking. Before long they were so wobbly that he couldn't sign his name or hold a cup. It took two hands to steady a spoon, but even then the spoon's contents ended up on his lap. His wife cut his food, and he drank coffee with a straw. He spent more time home, alone.

Medicines didn't work. "I am an avid golfer," Long told the FDA committee. "You can imagine. It is kind of difficult to have four putts on every green. I was fast becoming a hermit because I was too embarrassed to go out."

Long's case was so severe that his neurologist sent him for an evaluation at Kansas University Medical Center. In May 1996, neurosurgeon Steve Wilkinson and his team implanted electrodes deep in the left side of Long's brain. They also put a battery-powered control device in his chest wall. Two hours after the operation, Long was eating peas with a fork. The tremor in his right hand was gone. Six months later, neurosurgeons implanted electrodes on the right side of his brain. That day, he brought a cup of coffee to his lips and took his first gulp in years. He didn't need a straw.

"I eat soup for the first time in fourteen years. I can drink coffee from a cup. I go out. I can meet in the public and be happy and enjoy life," Long told the panel. "One good thing about this type of surgery and the implant is you can turn it on and off," Long added, as he demonstrated with a swipe of a handheld magnet across his chest. His hands immediately began to shake. A second swipe of the magnet turned the stimulator on again, and the tremor vanished after several seconds. "It is great. You can go to the golf course, have your device off, get on the putting green and get all the bets made, and then turn it on."

George Shafer, who flew up from Florida, told a similar story. His Parkinson's tremor made it impossible to button his shirts or to tie his shoes. Like Long, he would splatter food on the floor when he tried to eat without help. "I was a salesman for a food-service company. I would go out to meet a customer and I got a bad hand shaking and tremor, and I couldn't sell the product. You can't sell while shaking in front of somebody and give them confidence. After the operation, I was like a new man. I even made a model airplane to see if I could do it, small intricate work. After that, I made three or four candlestick holders. I still have Parkinson's, but I say I have got 50 percent of it beat."

In 1993, when Shafer had the electrodes implanted by surgeons at the University of South Florida, he became one of the first people in the United States to bear witness to the life-changing benefits of the device. "I say if there is anybody that should be a judge, or could be a judge, on whether it is needed or not, I don't know of any other one better than I am," Shafer said. "It is a wonderful miracle."

As on other FDA advisory panels, the voting members—all medical doctors or scientists with some expertise in the area being discussed— would decide whether or not to recommend that the FDA approve DBS. Internal teams at the FDA would then review the committee's recommendation. On March 14, the committee members listened to a few more testimonials, asked questions, and discussed the findings from the trial. They agreed that the study proved that deep brain stimulation was safe and effective for the treatment of essential tremor or Parkinson's tremor.[1] Six months later, in early August, the FDA approved the use of implanted brain stimulators to control tremors. They were approved for use on only one side of the brain at a time, in an area called the thalamus. (Studies on bilateral stimulation were still in the works.) And only Parkinson's patients with severe tremor could qualify for the procedure.

By 2008, 40,000 people around the world had had electrodes implanted in their brains to stimulate abnormal circuits, mostly to relieve Parkinson's disease and tremor. People afflicted with the violent involuntary muscle contractions of dystonia also had joined the ranks, and many hundreds of patients with disabling forms of other disorders—ranging from epilepsy to obsessive-compulsive disorder to Tourette syndrome—were receiving the treatment experimentally. For those enrolled in early, disease-specific trials of deep brain stimulation, the results were clearly encouraging. Data suggested that the human brain responds to the electrical signals and that the procedure can lead to significant improvement in a range of symptoms. Today, scientists are speculating that putting electrodes in the right spot in the brain might relieve chronic pain, ease intractable depression, enhance memory, alleviate chronic and debilitating headaches, and even help people lose weight.

This book tells the story of how deep brain stimulation unfolded as a potential therapy for many disparate brain diseases. It is a tale of successes, failures, and life somewhere in the middle of all this technology. It's about the science of brain circuitry. It's also about the scientists who are fighting to study this surgical technique in the right way—and with the right patients—to make sure that deep brain stimulation is not abused as a treatment. If the studies are not done right, it could mean the end of a potentially important tool to alleviate human suffering. This book is about some of the patients who have braved DBS surgeries and who walk around with electrodes in their brains and batteries in their chests as they benefit from the technology and yet remain aware that it could fail them. And finally, this book is a story about how research translates into a technology that has the potential to help people regain lives made grueling by illness. It is about hope and caution.

Part One

Parkinson's Disease: The Mother Lode

Chapter 1

Breaking Ground
100 Years of Research

B y the end of the twentieth century, Parkinson's disease was one of the best-studied disorders of the brain; researchers knew more about this affliction of movement than almost any other neurological or psychological disorder. Even though its cause remained unclear and its cure out of reach, a century of scientific efforts to treat Parkinson's became the research mother lode from which scientists mined and refined deep brain stimulation and began spreading its use worldwide.

Parkinson's disease has deep roots in medical history. The condition, which is marked by shaking, rigidity, and abnormal gait, appears in text written in 5000 BC. For centuries it was known as the "shaking palsy," a term first used by Galen in AD 164. A London physician, James Parkinson, formally described the disease in an 1817 essay that received little notice until 1861, when the French neurologist Jean-Martin Charcot drew attention to it, supplemented the list of symptoms, and named the disease after Parkinson. (Charcot also wrote about claims for cures using "electrotherapy" in the 1850s, but well-known physicians who experimented with these treatments in the late nineteenth century concluded that any benefit was psychological.)

What Parkinson described was people with severe tremors and other movement problems that grew worse over time. The symptoms of the disease emerge after a group of cells in the substantia nigra, an important movement-related structure in the midbrain, begins to die. These cells make a chemical called dopamine that is intimately tied to movement, coordination, and behavior. Today, more than a million people in the United States have Parkinson's. In addition to experiencing movement problems, many patients suffer cognitive deficits as well. Several medicines and surgical approaches are able to reduce the symptoms, but none stops the disease in its tracks.

Charcot studied and reported on patients with Parkinson's for almost twenty years. Other leading physicians joined Charcot in the race to unravel the puzzle of this movement disorder. The brain structures that would become key in the disease's treatment were the corpora striata, which today are known as the basal ganglia. From the 1870s to the 1920s, researchers developed persuasive evidence that diseased tissue in the substantia nigra was associated with Parkinson's pathology. The evidence arrived on the autopsy table, which was the only window into the brain at the time. Treatment for living sufferers would remain elusive until investigators could find a way to determine what the basal ganglia did and how they were involved with Parkinson's.

Only after neurosurgeons began using electrodes for brain mapping did some of the first insights into the Parkinson's pathological process begin to emerge. And with these findings came the first chance to do something about the disease. Thus, in the 1940s, a path of hope for patients began to appear. It started in neurosurgery and moved to medication, back to surgery, and ultimately to a unique way to silence abnormal cells—deep brain stimulation.[2]

The first documented meeting between electrode and brain actually took place in the 1870s, when British physician Richard Caton used a reflecting galvanometer to detect electrical currents in the exposed brains of rabbits and monkeys. The galvanometer, which consisted of a wire and coil, was named for Luigi Galvani, who in 1791 discovered electrical properties in human tissue. Caton believed that through his experiments, he had captured the physiological essence of a thought: "If I showed the monkey a raisin, but did not give it, a slight negative variation of the current occurred," he wrote.

As the years wore on, electrodes were developed as a way to detect brain waves through the human skull. In the early 1930s, a few researchers in the United States and Europe began to create brain maps by using electrical probes to stimulate different parts of the brains of animals and then recording changes in their movement or behavior.[3] But it was an American neurosurgeon working in Canada, Wilder Penfield, who in 1934 first brought electrodes to humans to map the brain.

Wilder Penfield was born in Spokane, Washington, in 1891. He studied at Princeton before winning a Rhodes scholarship to Oxford University. At Oxford, he pursued research in neuropathology under Sir Charles Scott Sherrington, a pathologist who arrived at Oxford in 1913. Sherrington mentored a handful of Rhodes scholars like Penfield and also planted the seeds of science in three students who went on to win the Nobel Prize. Penfield became interested in the nervous system, and he was especially focused on a condition called epilepsy.

Penfield moved to Canada early in his career and in 1934 established the Montreal Neurological Institute. At the hospital, he developed a neurosurgical procedure to eliminate seizures in epilepsy patients, and it became widely known as the Montreal Procedure. He administered a local anesthetic that allowed him to cut through the scalp and skull while patients remained conscious. Keeping the patient awake to express the activity in the brain centers was key, he thought, to guiding a surgeon. The brain is full of so many critical areas that regulate motion, mood, and sensory and cognitive processes that surgeons need to see and hear the patient's responses to know if they are entering risky terrain. Penfield also wanted to know when he reached the area of the seizure activity so that he could remove the brain tissue that was causing the seizures. The technique's use spread, as more than half of patients undergoing the Montreal Procedure were cured of their seizures.

In the operating room, with his epilepsy patients awake, Penfield applied electric currents to the surface of their brains to identify areas of high seizure activity. He wanted to see whether stimulation with electrodes could trigger the "aura" that patients said they experienced right before their seizures took hold. To his surprise, stimulating one area of the brain led to memories that seemed as real in the operating room as they had at the time of the initial experience. These memories had nothing to do with the seizures. His patients described sounds, colors, and movements. As he stimulated one region, a hand moved, or a leg, or the lid of an eye. Slowly, Penfield created what became known as the motor homunculus—the brain's own map of the entire human body during movement. In time, other brain explorers would discover similar homunculi in smaller brain targets, such as the subthalamic nucleus, the globus pallidus, and the thalamus.

By the 1940s Penfield's maps of the brain were guiding neurosurgeons into regions where none had dared travel before. Years of laboratory research on postmortem human and animal brains had yielded good ideas about where many disorders might originate, and neurosurgeons wanted to identify these abnormal regions to alleviate suffering in their patients. Unfortunately, they were without the luxury of modern CT or MRI scanning devices. Surgeons relied on crude mapping coordinates, metal-framed gear to position the head, and stereotactic techniques to navigate deep into the brain.

Stereotaxis helped, but it wasn't a perfect solution for explorations into the brain. One classic study showed that neurosurgeons guided by stereotaxis toward the thalamus ended up detouring to the pallidum. And even when they reached the right bit of tissue, so little was known about the pathophysiology of disease that it hardly mattered. For many brain diseases, experts tending to the brain didn't know where or what the problem was. It was a surgical guessing game.

But for the neurosurgeons trying to relieve Parkinson's and other movement disorders, it was helpful to know more exact locations of specific brain regions thought to be involved in movement. This knowledge allowed them to begin making small lesions in those areas of the brain. The basal ganglia and the thalamus had already been targeted as areas involved in Parkinson's, and thus those were the regions that neurosurgeons were trying to reach. But it was a "lesion and look" approach (damaging the area and looking for the effects), and generations of patients emerged from the operating room with inconsistent results.

Before stereotactic frames became available, many surgeons developed their own makeshift devices. Because the brain was closed, neurosurgeons would use external landmarks, measuring from the outside of the eye to the small projection at the bottom of the ear called the tragus. These external landmarks helped surgeons approximate the location of internal structures such as the anterior commissure (AC) and the posterior commissure (PC), two separate bundles of white matter fibers that pass in front of and behind the thalamus in the middle of the brain. These white matter tracts connect the different sides of the brain. Thus, by drawing a line from the middle of the AC to the middle of the PC, you get a route that connects front to back inside the brain. This route is considered the midline. Most brain structures are identified based on their location relative to this line or to its midpoint, called the midcommissural point.

Surgeons would then drill a hole in the brain and make their lesion based on the commissure roadway. "It was grossly inaccurate," said Jerrold Vitek, a neurologist who has been mapping the brain since his medical school days at the University of Minnesota in the 1970s.

Locating brain tissue remained virtually a guessing game until 1947, when neurologist Ernest A. Spiegel and neurosurgeon Henry T. Wycis of Temple University published a landmark paper in the journal *Science*. The paper described how an apparatus invented by British physicians Sir Victor A. H. Horsley and Robert H. Clarke for animal experiments could be used in humans.[4] This device, which would allow brain surgeons to reach specific targets more accurately as they headed into the brain, used a three-dimensional coordinate system based on specific anatomical landmarks in the brain relative to a frame that was anchored to the skull.

The apparatus that Spiegel and Wycis developed would change the course of neurosurgery. They put their patients into the head frame, bolted the patient's skull into the device, and created a three-dimensional model of the internal structures in the brain. "That brought us closer to the target, but individual brains vary enough that it still wasn't an exact surgical procedure," said Vitek.

Two years after Spiegel and Wycis introduced their head frame, a Swedish neurosurgeon named Lars Leksell introduced his own apparatus, which was brought into the neurosurgical operating room.[5] Instead of using the Cartesian coordinates that Horsley and Clarke had developed for animal studies, Leksell relied on polar coordinates, a system in which each point on a plane is determined by both an angle and a distance. By contrast, Cartesian coordinates consist of two perpendicular lines crossing at a central point; a position, or coordinate, is determined according to its east-west and north-south displacement from the lines.

Leksell used his stereotactic frame to conduct experiments on patients with Parkinson's disease. Many neurosurgeons of the day followed suit. Leksell knew that he wanted to make a lesion in the basal ganglia, but the structures were rather large. They consisted of distinct substructures, including the caudate nucleus, the putamen, the globus pallidus, and the subthalamic nucleus. So, throughout the 1950s, Leksell made lesions going from the front of the basal ganglia to the back. He discovered that the patients who showed the most improvement had lesions in the posterior lateral portion of the internal segment of the globus pallidus.

In 1960, Leksell and his colleague E. Svennilson published a paper in a European journal. They described surgeries on eighty-one Parkinson's patients. Nineteen of the twenty patients who had lesions in the posterior portion of the globus pallidus (the internal segment) had the best response.[6] The procedure, called a pallidotomy, helped reduce tremors, rigidity, and slowness of movement in the patients. Leksell and Svennilson's report was a landmark in the treatment of Parkinson's. But the significance of their discovery was not as clear then as it would become two decades later. At the time, it simply joined the small body of literature informing the neurosurgeons who were quietly building an understanding of how to use surgery in the brain for movement disorders—quietly, that is, except for one.

Chapter 2

Coop the King

Controversy on the Frontier

In 1954, a German neurology journal published a study by an anatomist named Rolf Hassler, who had tried lesioning the thalamus of Parkinson's patients and had observed that tremor was reduced dramatically.[7] While pallidotomy produced more global effects on Parkinson's symptoms, thalamotomy had such a more immediate and dramatic effect on tremor that it was to become the surgery of choice for the next decade. During that time, surgeons tried different targets in the thalamus until they found one that worked best: the ventral intermediate (VIM) nucleus. Decades later, Finnish neurosurgeon Lauri Laitinen would publish a paper on the large discrepancy between targets across surgeons. Historically, some surgeons trying to land on the thalamus would consider it a success to reach the anterior of the VIM, while others would be happy reaching just below the thalamus itself. But in New York, one young neurosurgeon learned of Hassler's report and was impressed. Without hesitation, he added thalamotomy to his repertoire of procedures.

Brazen in the operating room and brash in the media, Irving S. Cooper was the sort of clinical scientist who put others in the field on edge. Scientists, then and now, hate hype, especially when it comes to new and unproven medical findings. The hoopla inevitably raises false, or at least premature, hopes and depletes the public's patience with the slow, careful scientific studies and replication of findings that lie at the heart of real progress in science. Thus many researchers bristled as Cooper aggressively promoted his results, both to the research world and to the public at large. He even showed movies of his dramatically recovered patients. Fellow researchers blanched as he pulled neurosurgery out of its quiet, meticulous obscurity and gave it a noisy boot into the mainstream.

But Cooper was talented, and when all was said and done, he was a pioneer in the early surgical management of movement disorders. He used a variety of surgical techniques, including innovations of his own, to operate on some of the worst cases of movement disorders in the world. And it was hard to gauge his success. In 1960, a thirty-eight-year-old Cooper published findings from his surgeries for Parkinson's and other movement disorders using pallidotomy and thalamotomy, most of which he said were successful and free of serious complications.

In all, Cooper reportedly operated on more than five thousand Parkinson's patients. During his career, he used not only the scalpel to lesion brain tissue but also chemicals and freezing, and in the 1970s he enlisted engineers to help him design one of the earliest deep brain stimulation devices. He used this device to treat intractable spasticity and seizures in some of his patients and, in the first study on deep brain stimulation in humans ever to be published in a scientific journal, reported that 55 percent of the patients improved. His colleagues of the day may not have been impressed by his purported successes, but four decades later, a new generation of neurosurgeons looked back on his work with reverence. In 1998, a team of surgeons wrote a paper on Irving S. Cooper. They called him a pioneer in functional neurosurgery.[8]

Irving Cooper was born on July 15, 1922. He received his doctorate in medicine from George Washington University in 1945 and enlisted in the U.S. Navy. He served an internship at the United States Naval Hospital in 1946, and later in his enlistment, at a base near the Arabian Peninsula, he doctored soldiers who had been wounded in the Korean War. Cooper was tall, blond, athletic, and self-confident. With his knack for languages, he could present lectures in Japanese and read operas in Italian. After his service in the navy, Cooper completed his neurosurgical training at the Mayo Clinic in Rochester, Minnesota, in 1951, but he was eager to join the ranks of New York neurosurgeons. He landed a position in the department of neurosurgery at New York University, which had been officially inaugurated only a year earlier.

Early on, Cooper was interested in the surgical procedures being developed for patients with movement disorders. Operations for these patients had been going on for more than a dozen years, mainly on Parkinson's patients, and surgeons had tried many targets in the brain. When Cooper entered the NYU operating suite, the procedure of choice was pedunculotomy, a cut of the pyramidal tract in the midbrain. Other neurosurgeons, however, were cutting tissue in the globus pallidus and the ansa lenticularis to alleviate rigidity and tremor.

Ten years earlier, in 1942, in a cautionary example of the hazards in operating on the brain, a Chicago neurosurgeon named Paul Bucy had reported that some Parkinson's patients were emerging from surgery with partial paralysis. He had been targeting their brains' premotor and motor cortex areas. Though the tremors were gone, the patients were left with severe weakness, even paralysis, on one side of the body. The operation also triggered seizures, thus leading Bucy to the conclusion that such operations should not be done. Bucy's experience made it into surgical textbooks and helped shift the neurosurgical focus to targets within the basal ganglia and thalamus. But still, a scientific review published in 1951 quoted one of Bucy's colleagues, Chicago's Dr. Roland Mackay, as saying that "neurosurgical procedures had no place in the treatment of the vast problems of involuntary movement disorders."

Irving Cooper was obviously not going by the textbooks of his day. In October 1951, he was operating on a Parkinson's patient with violent resting tremor. He made his way to the same motor fibers that Bucy had warned against lesioning. However, before he reached the motor fiber, he nicked a small artery at the base of the man's brain. It was serious. The man could have bled to death, and so Cooper used tiny silver clips to ligate the artery. The surgery was aborted. Cooper replaced the bone flaps, closed the scalp, and called it a bad day.

When the patient awoke from the anesthesia, the tremors on the left side of his body were gone. (The right side of the brain controls the left side of the body, and the left brain commands the right side.) Cooper had made a movie of his patient before and after the surgery, and he showed it to colleagues. "It is impressive but a long way from proving anything," Fred Mettler, a professor of anatomy at Columbia University, told him. Mettler, whose experience was limited to animals with involuntary movement disorders, invited Cooper to come uptown to Columbia and operate on some chimps in his laboratory. Cooper accepted. His first patient was Rosebud. After she was anesthetized, Cooper opened her brain and cut the same artery he had nicked accidentally in the surgery on his patient. Mettler conducted the autopsy of Rosebud's brain. The artery blockage had deprived oxygen and had quite specifically damaged areas of the basal ganglia, an area where abnormalities were known to be involved in movement disorders.

Cooper became a regular visitor at the NYU hospital morgue. When he heard the code "special conference" announced over the hospital loud-speakers, it meant an autopsy was under way in the basement. When permission was granted, Cooper took some of the patient's brain tissue for study. He cut the artery. He found that its path led to the thalamus, a nearby region called the internal capsule, and sometimes the globus pallidus.

Cooper had been following the established procedure, pedunculotomy, targeting the pyramidal tract in the midbrain, but he wanted to go after the anterior choroidal artery—the one he had accidentally nicked. Cooper found a patient for his surgical experiment: a thirty-six-year-old man named Raymond Walker in a psychiatric hospital on Long Island. They met in the winter of 1951.

Walker, at age nineteen, had been admitted to a New York hospital unconscious, delirious, and with a spiking fever. The doctors' diagnosis was von Economo's encephalitis, or sleeping sickness. A virus had made its way into Walker's brain. When he regained consciousness weeks later, he had such violent tremors, even as his muscles remained rigid, that he could no longer control his limbs. His words came out in a whisper, if at all. His face had lost its expression.

With his tremors advancing, Walker had been shuttled from one hospital to the next until he ended up in the hands of a psychoanalyst. It was noted in his thick medical chart that on rare occasions the rigidity and motionlessness would spontaneously disappear. For those few moments Walker could talk, but he was so angry about the state of his "dying body," as he told the analyst, that he no longer wanted to live. During one of these brief passages of control, he rammed his head through a window and shook it back and forth hoping that the shards of glass would sever the arteries in his neck. That was how he had ended up at Central Islip Psychiatric Hospital on Long Island. He spent his days motionless, speechless, and tethered to a bed.

In Cooper's 1981 autobiography, *Vital Probe*, he wrote of Raymond Walker: "His uncontrollably trembling muscles, paradoxically, were so stiff and rigid that he could not move them voluntarily. In constant motion, he could not choose to move himself. He was a frozen, songless wing-flapping bird confined to a constantly shaking cage." Walker was seven years older than Cooper, but the "songless" bird looked twice the age of his neurosurgeon. Cooper proposed a possible cure: cutting the anterior choroidal artery. Walker's sister, his only living relative, agreed to the surgery. It took place in February 1952.

Cooper used an electrical current to cauterize the artery. After the surgery, the left side of Raymond's body continued to jerk violently. The right side was quiet, however, and his movement, for the first time in almost eighteen years, was under his command. Cooper wrote in his autobiography of the outcome: "There was nothing that could be said that would surpass the expression or the significance of Raymond's fingers snapping."

That night, Cooper was settled in for the evening when a call from the hospital reported that Walker had lost consciousness. Cooper rushed back to the hospital. Walker was already primed for surgery. When he opened up the skull, Cooper found the problem. It was a brain hemorrhage. He stopped the bleeding and cleared the area. Three days later Walker was snapping his fingers again and eating his meals with his own hands. On the fifth day, he stood on his own and walked out of the recovery room. And for the next few days the nurses watched as he walked to the Coca Cola vending machine and used his right hand to place a nickel into the thin slot and grab a bottle. The nurses were happy to provide the nickels. For ten consecutive days, he made more than fifty trips to the soda machine, each time downing the contents of the glass bottle in a single gulp.

A month later, in March 1952, Cooper took Walker back into the operating room to occlude the artery on the other side of his brain. When the tremors continued, Cooper injected dye into the artery and used a crude scanning device to evaluate the situation. The small artery was still open. Walker was taken back to surgery. This was his fourth surgical trip in a span of two months, but Walker didn't seem to care. In mid-April of that year, two weeks after his last surgery, the once-mute and immobile man was on the floor doing twenty-five consecutive push-ups to demonstrate the strength and control of his body. In June, he walked out of the state psychiatric hospital and into a new life.

In the year after he operated on Walker, Cooper followed with surgeries on eleven more patients with intractable tremors and rigidity. Six improved, four didn't, and one died. But Cooper talked only about the successes. He would go to medical meetings and show movies of Walker and the others before and after surgery. He also sent a report on his neurosurgery techniques to the American Neurological Association. A professor of neurology at Columbia, Dr. H. Houston Merritt, invited him to give a ten-minute talk at the association's 1953 annual meeting in Atlantic City.

The thirty-two-year-old neurosurgeon was the first speaker on the long agenda. Technicians threaded a reel of his movie footage onto the projector, and, after his talk, a hundred of Cooper's colleagues watched Raymond Walker transform from a mute and trembling victim to a man easily doing twenty-five push-ups. William Laurence, a reporter for the *New York Times*, was in the audience. His story on Cooper was in the next day's newspaper.

Despite Cooper's promotion of his procedure, the results of the anterior choroidal artery surgery proved inconsistent. As a few other surgeons also were starting to do, he began to target the basal ganglia, which was the same area damaged in Rosebud the chimp's brain.

Then, in 1954, Cooper made a career move. The Home for the Incurables, which had opened in the Bronx a year after the Civil War ended, had been the first chronic disease hospital in the country. Now called St. Barnabas Hospital, it was bursting with patients with chronic and intractable movement disorders. The owners offered Cooper three operating rooms of his own. The hospital sat on a beautiful hill in an Italian neighborhood with markets and restaurants, where Cooper could practice his love of the Italian language.

Cooper's operating rooms were laboratories where he would develop new techniques to stop abnormal movements. He would not only operate on Parkinson's patients but also begin taking on the movement problems of children with dystonia (a disorder that causes uncontrollable muscle contractions), cerebral palsy, and epilepsy. He also took pain patients into his operating rooms. He would damage the abnormal tissue by dripping alcohol onto his target—an approach he called chemopallidectomy or chemothalamectomy, depending on where he was aiming. He would go on to publish several reports, even books, on these procedures.[9]

The work was decidedly controversial. Cooper was seen as a maverick, a cowboy. While other neurosurgeons were slowly marking the road to treatments for movement disorders, Cooper was the guy blowing the loudest horn. Many of his contemporaries found his style abrasive, and they worried that he never seemed to have any failures emerge from his operating room.

Dr. Paul Bucy, the Illinois neurosurgeon who had urged against such operations, stood up at a medical meeting and referred to Cooper's work as "ballyhoo," according to Cooper's account in his autobiography.

Cooper's wife, Sissel, remembered a different Coop, a man who cared passionately about his patients and was a maverick, not a cowboy—and certainly someone who "was ahead of his time." She said that he knew he couldn't cure everybody, although he might have liked to, and actually turned many patients away. In later years, he started a foundation to support medicine and the humanities because, she said, "he felt that medicine had lost a lot of its compassion for the patient."

Although Cooper was controversial, in 1959, when he was thirty-seven, he was respected enough to be invited to the prestigious Johns Hopkins Medical Institutes to give a talk. But while he was at a chalkboard in a room filled with doctors, a neurologist named Charles Luttrell walked in and declared, "I am here to say that your work is a known fraud. The American Medical Association should see to it that people like you are not allowed to practice. This whole thing has been a pack of lies, about Parkinsonism and all the rest."

Such comments failed to discourage Cooper. He kept looking for innovative ways to treat the hardest cases. According to his wife, one of his ideas was inspired by a Christmas present. He had received a corkscrew filled with liquid nitrogen, and during one of his first tries at opening a bottle of wine he stuck himself with the needle at the end of the corkscrew. Liquid nitrogen temporarily froze his finger. He wondered if he could develop an instrument that would release a freezing agent into the brain to cool the tissue. With help from an engineer, Cooper designed the first cryosurgical (freezing) probe for neurosurgical patients. His first cryosurgery was performed in 1961. Cooper also began operating on the internal capsule and thalamus of epilepsy and dystonia patients. Many of his colleagues challenged his claims that the patients were virtually cured, but patients didn't care. They would do anything to get control of their bodies.

Life magazine photographer Margaret Bourke-White was diagnosed with Parkinson's in 1956. Three years later, Cooper performed brain surgery on her while a photographer took pictures of the entire operation. The surgery was successful. It controlled her tremors and enabled her to return to work. *Life* published a story on her surgery, complete with pictures of Cooper,[10] and Bourke-White's neurosurgeon gained immediate acclaim. But her symptoms returned in 1961. Another round in Cooper's operating room didn't help. In fact, it triggered some speech problems.

When Cooper learned about the work of his friend George C. Cotzias, who developed L-dopa as the first medicine for Parkinson's in 1961, he reportedly deferred seven hundred scheduled surgeries and enrolled the patients in levodopa clinical trials at St. Barnabas. Cooper said he would stop accepting patients into his operating room if medicines could do the trick.

In the pre L-dopa days, Cooper operated on as many as six patients a day. Once L-dopa became available to Parkinson's patients, he averaged only two a day. But they tended to be patients that no one else would take or that were offered little help by other doctors. They came from all over the country and from overseas.

Coop the King was what Patricia Kabram called Cooper, mostly in admiration but also with a nod to his famous ego. Kabram had found her way to Cooper in search of help for her eight-year-old daughter, Lisa, who had developed dystonia when she was four. The little girl's limbs were always in motion; she had constant spasms in her back, and she couldn't bend at the waist.

Cooper ended up operating on Lisa seven times. With each surgery, she got a little better, but never well enough to stand on her own. Finally, the little girl who could only crawl was able to sit up in a wheelchair. Though she had difficulty speaking and remained in a wheelchair, Lisa graduated from high school and completed a year of college. Disabled but not dispirited, she worked her way into voluntary and then paying jobs.

Lisa's mother, meanwhile, started having back spasms of her own when she was thirty-seven. Previously, her symptoms had always been mild; poor penmanship was her biggest problem. When Patricia was in college, doctors thought her symptoms were psychological because she could write the word *daddy* in big letters but not in small ones. Her father also had problems writing, but nothing much was made of this odd fact. Then Kabram learned that some forms of dystonia were genetic. She had inherited it from her father and had passed it on to Lisa.

Before Cooper operated on Patricia Kabram in 1973, she could no longer cut her food, and she had such horrible back spasms that she could be thrown to the ground when standing on both feet. Following the surgery, she was served chicken and cut it herself with her right hand. The scooter that had helped her get around gathered dust in a corner of her house. She was walking again. But whatever improvement Cooper's surgery brought, it was temporary for both mother and daughter. Their symptoms worsened over time.

Lisa and Patricia tried every experimental therapy for dystonia. Finally, in 2007, Patricia had electrodes implanted in her brain and a battery pack inserted in her chest wall. Lisa also had had deep brain stimulation surgery a few years earlier, but the surgeons at Mount Sinai Medical Center had said that Lisa's brain was already so scarred from many operations that it was doubtful the stimulators would work. They were right. Two years after her deep brain stimulation surgery, pneumonia delivered the final blow to Lisa's body. She was forty-five.

Another of Cooper's patients was Margaret Dever. Born in 1946 with mild cerebral palsy, she was always in regular classes at school, but in 1965, in her second semester of college, she developed severe pain in her right hip. She couldn't walk. Doctors put her in a chest cast and used a new drug called Valium to calm her muscles. "My right arm was bent like a pretzel," Dever recalled. Doctors sent her to the Rusk Institute in New York for three months. In New York, her parents learned about Irving S. Cooper.

On July 15, 1965, Cooper used his cryosurgical technique to freeze a part of Dever's thalamus, on the left side of her brain. A nurse asked Dever, who was wide awake during the surgery, to touch her nose with her right finger. "I can't do that," she said. "My right hand is uncontrollable." But she held up her right hand and smoothly reached down to touch her nose. "Oh, my God," she kept saying, as she moved her steady right hand at arm's length and then brought it back to her nose. Cooper saw Dever every three months for two years. "He wanted to take me to Russia and Finland to show people my progress. I said no, I had final exams to take," said Dever.

But patients like Margaret Dever were balanced by others like Frank Greco, a thirty-nine-year-old postal worker who suffered permanent brain damage after undergoing one of Cooper's surgeries in 1970. Greco spent the rest of his life in a nursing home, and his family sued. Nine years after the surgery, Greco was awarded $1.8 million, a record for a personal-injury case in New York State at the time. (The award was assessed against Cooper and another physician, Dr. Joseph Walz, as well as St. Barnabas Hospital.)[11]

By the time the suit was settled, Cooper was on the downside of his career. He was working at a Westchester County hospital, as well as devoting time to writing books for both doctors and patients. He even wrote a novel about the life of a patient with neurological disease. In the book, *It's Hard to Leave When the Music's Playing*, a neurosurgeon helps a friend with amyotrophic lateral sclerosis (ALS, also called Lou Gehrig's disease) end his life. Cooper himself died of lung cancer in 1985. He was sixty-three.[12]

Chapter 3

Finding the
Parkinson's Problem

The basal ganglia are a collection of gray matter structures connected by fibers (the brain's white matter tracts) to each other and to a family of circuits in the cerebral cortex. The basal ganglia, along with another large chunk of tissue in the back of the brain called the cerebellum, are part of a complex network of cells that modulate—that is, adjust through exciting or inhibiting—movement, emotions, and cognitive processes around the clock.

The cortex has direct connections to the thalamus, as well as to the striatum of the basal ganglia. All three structures modulate movement, but the relationships among them remain unclear. The strongest direct projections are from the basal ganglia and the cerebellum to the thalamus; from the thalamus to the cortex; and from the cortex to the thalamus and the basal ganglia.

Neurons in these structures are filled with chemicals and electrical signals that provide a complex communication system between various brain regions. The basal ganglia are thought to support movement by modulating neuronal activity in different regions of the brain. The work of the basal ganglia, along with other motor structures, allows people to make smooth movements at their own pace and with the will of their thoughts.

People with movement disorders have abnormal networks. The firing of the cells—and the excitation and inhibition that take place in the basal ganglia—are off-kilter, and the result is uncontrolled movement. For Parkinson's patients, this imbalance causes tremors, rigid muscles, an unsteady gait, and often an inability to move at will. Patients may freeze in place. Dystonia patients, on the other hand, suffer from uncontrollable involuntary movements that can become worse when the patient moves. The strength of the missed basal ganglia signals can throw some people to the floor and cause their limbs to writhe so wildly that restraint is necessary.

The basal ganglia are like a neighborhood in the brain. The names of the neighborhood's buildings are caudate, putamen, globus pallidus, substantia nigra, and nucleus accumbens. The fibers heading in and out of these structures are like the streets. Another neighborhood that borders on the basal ganglia has a group of interconnected structures often called the limbic system (this term has fallen out of favor with brain researchers). The important limbic structures are the thalamus, the amygdala, the hippocampus, and the hypothalamus. Along with the cortex, the basal ganglia are key structures in developing goal-directed and motivated behaviors. They are also involved in the regulation of mood.

The early pioneers who set out to understand the brain tried structure after structure in the neighborhood of the basal ganglia until they found the ones that would alleviate the symptoms of movement disorders. The neurosurgeons who began operating on these patients in the 1940s were destroying what they hoped was abnormal tissue. But there was scant scientific proof to justify their techniques and treatments, which they developed more or less by accident. Someone tried something; it worked; others began doing it. At the same time, scientists began to study the brain's inner workings systematically. They started the painstaking work of figuring out what exactly was taking place inside this three-pound tissue.

In time, and fortunately, neurosurgeons began working alongside neurologists and scientists. Taking a leaf from Wilder Penfield's book, they began using stimulating electrodes to guide them to specific brain tissue. The move to use this tool during surgery was what eventually led surgeons to leave the electrodes in place.

By the late 1950s, Arvid Carlsson, a Swedish researcher and physician, had identified dopamine in the brain and had figured out a way to measure dopamine levels in the basal ganglia. (Carlsson's work led to a shared Nobel Prize in physiology or medicine in 2000.) He showed that animals whose basal ganglia were depleted of dopamine developed the same abnormal movements as a Parkinson's patient. But restoring dopamine to the brain was a challenge, because the substance could not cross the blood-brain barrier—the tight mesh of cells in brain blood-vessel walls that keeps molecules in the blood from entering the brain.

Then George C. Cotzias, a neurologist and scientist who worked at Brookhaven National Laboratory on Long Island, developed a precursor of dopamine called L-dopa. He showed that L-dopa crossed into the brain and broke down to form the dopamine needed to restore levels of the chemical to the basal ganglia in Parkinson's patients. (In India five thousand years ago, the medical practice Ayurveda used a tropical pod called *Mucuna pruriens* to treat Parkinson's, then called kampavata. The seeds are a natural source of therapeutic quantities of L-dopa.[13])

Cotzias is best known for his L-dopa research, but that was not his only important work. He also studied trace metals in men who excavated manganese ore in Chilean mines. Some of them developed severe movement disorders, identical to what he had observed in Parkinson's patients. Cotzias discovered that a toxin in the ore damaged the substantia nigra, the same region hard hit in Parkinson's disease. This region was normally rich with dopamine, but in both cases—the miners' and the Parkinson's patients'—this neurotransmitter was depleted from the cells. Cotzias's report on these studies in 1966 was one of the earliest to suggest environmental triggers for the development of Parkinson's.

But if anyone deserves credit for unraveling the normal physiology of the basal ganglia, it is Mahlon DeLong, a neurologist whose laboratory interests gravitated naturally to his passion for treating patients with movement disorders. In the late 1970s, DeLong was also navigating the neurons of the basal ganglia, but instead of focusing so much on which neurons were abnormal in Parkinson's disease, he studied what the neurons might be doing in the first place. DeLong discovered that many different types of neurons populated this grape-size region and that these neurons were active in different ways.

DeLong graduated from Harvard Medical School in 1966 and joined the National Institute of Mental Health (NIMH) where he was introduced to the inner workings of the brain by Edward Vaughan Evarts, a neurophysiologist. Evarts had devised a way to record individual neurons in the brains of monkeys as they carried out a variety of tasks. Evarts was especially interested in the motor cortex. When he began studying the basal ganglia, scientists thought that they were pathways that funneled commands to the cortex from different cortical areas.

Using Evarts's tools to study the activity of basal ganglia neurons in primates, DeLong characterized the properties of these regions. He focused on comparisons between basal ganglia neurons and neurons in the cerebellum and motor cortex, studies that were being carried out by Tom Thach and Evarts.

DeLong spent five years in Evarts's laboratory before beginning a neurology residency at Johns Hopkins in 1973. During his residency, he began seeing patients with movement disorders. After his residency, he joined the Hopkins faculty, and he continued his research to unravel the puzzles of basal ganglia structure and function, as well as the basis of Parkinson's and other disorders of the basal ganglia.

The research that emerged from DeLong's lab—led by Peter Strick, whose brilliant anatomical studies helped define the region—indicated that the basal ganglia were actually part of parallel and separate pathways. They were closed loops with a route that began in specific areas of the cortex and returned home through the basal ganglia and the thalamus. These included motor, oculomotor, limbic, and associative circuits. This discovery made it possible to understand how abnormalities in these discrete circuits, caused by damage to the structures, could lead to a broad range of problems. To DeLong and his collaborators, it was a huge breakthrough in understanding how the basal ganglia caused disturbances of movement, mood, and behavior.

At Hopkins, DeLong, Gary Alexander, and Strick described the basal ganglia pathway in the normal brains of monkeys. Another colleague,

Apostolos Georgopoulos, worked on the basic physiology of the basal ganglia and the subthalamic nucleus. The subthalamic nucleus would get its day in the sun because of an unfortunate series of events in California that would change the trajectory of Parkinson's research forever.

In 1982, men and women began showing up in emergency rooms unable to move or speak. They were young and frozen. It would take a bit of detective work by California neurologist Dr. J. William Langston to figure out what was going on.[14]

These people had something in common: they had all recently injected bad heroin. Langston got hold of some samples, but his chemists could not figure out what it was. They knew what it wasn't. It was not heroin. At the same time, police in San Jose, California, were also interested in having the "heroin" samples analyzed. A crime unit chemist, Halle Weingarten, ran a sample and thought it might be a close match to a drug she had seen before: meperidine, an opioid painkiller commonly known as Demerol. Weingarten remembered that in the journal *Psychiatry Research* she had read about a case of an addict who developed a similarly bizarre freezing condition. When Langston called the next day to see if she had solved the mystery—what was the substance causing these paralyzing symptoms?—she sent the doctor to the journal article.

The journal was obscure, and it soon became obvious why: the article in question was in the journal's first issue. It reported a case study of a college student who had used his chemistry set, a gift from his parents, to fashion a formula copied directly from a patent of a compound synthesized by a Hoffman-La Roche chemist in 1947. This compound—1-methyl-4-phe-nyl-4-propionoxy-piperidine, or MPPP—was an analog of meperidine. The Hoffman-La Roche chemist's analog was five times as potent as Demerol. The college student began making it and injecting it for a potent, heroin-like high. For several months in the summer of 1976, the student's chemistry lessons had been successful. Then, on one fateful day, the young man made a mistake with his chemical soup, and the injected contents burned as they coursed through his veins. Within three days, he was frozen.

At first, baffled doctors thought they were treating a case of catatonic schizophrenia, but when the drugs used for schizophrenia didn't work—and even electroshock therapy didn't help—a neurologist added up all the symptoms and diagnosed Parkinson's disease. He treated the young man with L-dopa, and his symptoms dramatically improved.

The young man was sent to the National Institutes of Health (NIH) so that doctors and scientists could figure out exactly what had happened. They were intrigued that he had somehow made a toxic substance that could trigger an acute and devastating Parkinson's-like syndrome. An NIMH chemist, Sanford Markey, was in charge of determining what went wrong in the young man's chemistry session. Luckily, the young man's parents were cooperative, and they invited Markey into the makeshift laboratory. There was a piece of glassware that had a small amount of residue, enough perhaps to identify the toxic substance the young "chemist" had inadvertently made. Markey took the sample back to the laboratory and used mass spectrometry to analyze its chemistry. It turned out to be a chemical called 1-methyl-4-phenyl-1,2,3,6-tetrahydropyridine, or MPTP. MPPP was also identified in the mix.

Two years after the young man injected MPTP, he was found dead under a tree on the NIH campus in Bethesda after overdosing on cocaine. His parents allowed an autopsy so that scientists could see what had gone wrong in their son's brain. Indeed, the area hard hit in Parkinson's, the substantia nigra, was literally destroyed. Any pathologist unfamiliar with the story would have looked at the autopsy slides and diagnosed Parkinson's disease.[15]

With the paper in hand, Langston called Glen Davis, lead author of the study in *Psychiatry Research*. With new clues from Davis, Langston called Stanford University's Drug Assay Lab. He asked for chemist and lab director Ian Irwin. Irwin ticked off the formula for MPTP. It matched the atomic weight of the mysterious samples used by the frozen addicts in California.[16]

Once it became clear that MPTP was the chemical that had triggered sudden symptoms of the worst case of Parkinson's, scientists set out to test it in animals to see if it would have the same effect. If it did, could this chemical help determine what exactly was going wrong in the disease? The first to do these experiments was Stanley Burns, a neurologist in his thirties who was completing a fellowship at NIMH. His interest was the kinetics of the distribution of dopamine metabolites in monkeys. Burns had not been involved with the young drug addict who had accidentally made MPTP, but Irwin J. Kopin, chief of the Laboratory of Clinical Sciences at NIMH and a coauthor of the paper in *Psychiatry Research,* brought him into the fold to work the case of the frozen addicts in California.

In 1982, NIMH chemist Sandy Markey injected MPTP into rats. Nothing happened. Burns was not that surprised, since rodents respond to drugs differently than humans do. Markey had access to monkeys, however, and if MPTP was the toxin that induced Parkinson's, then a monkey might develop the same freezing symptoms that had felled the drug addicts. When Markey found the right dose, and gave it over several days, the monkey developed the same signs of Parkinson's. And L-dopa almost completely reversed the symptoms.

When the animal's brain was analyzed, the scientists could not find the substantia nigra; it had been totally destroyed. Stan Burns made history as the first to develop an animal model of Parkinson's disease. Scientists began using the MPTP model to understand Parkinson's. From the mid-1980s through the mid- to late 1990s, the first animal models of the disease led to new and more effective treatments. The field exploded with new information. This allowed scientists to move beyond Parkinson's to follow clues to other movement disorders. In particular, during the seven years from 1985 to 1992, lingering questions about the best place in the brain to treat Parkinson's began to be laid to rest.

At Johns Hopkins University, DeLong and William Miller, a physician working on a postdoctoral dissertation, were among the first scientists to record neuronal firing in the brains of monkeys injected with MPTP. In a 1987 report published in *Advances in Behavioral Biology,* they described changes in the activity of globus pallidus neurons. More specifically, they found that neurons in the internal segment of the globus pallidus, which give rise to the major output from the basal ganglia, were overactive.[17]

This was important news. The globus pallidus is made up of two parts, the internal segment and the external segment. What surgeons had learned from the early days of lesioning was that damage to the external segment causes worsening symptoms (which wasn't fully appreciated), while lesions to the internal segment—the motor posterolateral portion—are beneficial. The firing rates in these two segments are changed in patients with Parkinson's disease. Now DeLong and Miller had explained the changes.

Before DeLong and Miller's report, many Parkinson's researchers believed that both regions involved in the disease were *under*active because of the paucity of patients' movement and the difficulty they had initiating movement. The findings added a significant nuance: neural firing in the globus pallidus's external segment goes down, and activity in the internal segment goes up.

DeLong and Miller's finding would ultimately alter the landscape of Parkinson's treatment. DeLong, Hagai Bergman, and Thomas Wichmann demonstrated that the excess activity in the internal pallidum was a result of increased excitatory input from the subthalamic nucleus, a small structure known to cause involuntary movements when damaged. Then they showed that a lesion of the subthalamic nucleus in an afflicted monkey was effective in reducing the symptoms of Parkinson's disease. In 1990, the journal *Science* would publish DeLong's MPTP monkey work, including the benefits of reversing symptoms by chemically lesioning the subthalamic nucleus.[18]

Jerrold Vitek, who had spent a decade completing his medical and postdoctoral degrees at the University of Minnesota, chose Hopkins for his residency in neurology. Because of his strong research background (he studied the cerebellum), he quickly became one of DeLong's protégés. Arriving at Hopkins in 1984, Vitek began doing functional recordings of the motor region of the thalamus. The thalamus sits next to the ventricles in the middle of the brain and receives projections from the basal ganglia and the cerebellum. Both of these regions are intimately involved in movement. Vitek says that "nothing gets to the cortex unless it goes through the thalamus first."

In 1985, while DeLong and his colleagues were sorting out the mystery of the firing rates in the internal and external segments of the globus pallidus, Finnish neurosurgeon Lauri Laitinen reached into the past and rekindled surgical interest in that same structure, which had been a target in the pre-L-dopa decades of Parkinson's surgery. For more than two decades, Parkinson's patients had been relying on L-dopa to treat their symptoms, but the medicine was proving to have its own problems. Patients were experiencing "on and off" fluctuations as the medicine wore off during the day. They could be walking and moving about rather easily, but all of a sudden their bodies would become rigid as rock and they would freeze in place. It was no way to live. What's more, as dopamine cells in the brain continued to die away, the medicine had less effect. And in time doctors (and patients) realized that the medicine also had its own side effect. It could cause dyskinesia—wild, uncontrollable flailing movements.

Patients who were not doing well on L-dopa opted for surgery, which was still being offered around the world. But the surgical target was the thalamus, which was potent in stopping resting tremors but did little to help any of the other problems Parkinson's patients were living with. On January 30, 1985, Laitinen took a Parkinson's patient into surgery and ablated (destroyed) the pallidum on one side of her brain. For years she hadn't walked two steps without freezing or falling. Laitinen was taking a chance in reviving the old surgical procedure of Lars Leksell with modern-day tools. It worked. He went on to operate on another thirty-five patients and painstakingly followed them for years before submitting a paper on the results to the prestigious *Journal of Neurosurgery*.

The paper was rejected in 1990. The reviewers saw pallidotomy as an old technique that should have been kept where it belonged—in the past. Laitinen wrote directly to Thoralf Sundt, a neurosurgeon at the Mayo Clinic who was also the editor of the journal, and Sundt appreciated the work's importance. The study was published in 1992, and it became the single most-quoted paper in Parkinson's surgery.[19]

Pallidotomy made its comeback, but outcomes were not the same in all hands. Some surgeons headed too close to the midline near the internal capsule and got into trouble. Others went too deep and infringed on the optic tract, causing partial loss of vision. And still others headed too far to the anterior and produced cognitive problems. Even if they were close but not on target, surgeons might get a partial effect. But patients who couldn't swallow or speak were certainly not good for business.

The pace was picking up. Doctors and researchers were coming closer to figuring out the brain circuitry underlying Parkinson's disease. While Laitinen was revitalizing surgery for the disease, scientists following DeLong's lead were gaining more and more insight into the functional organization of the basal ganglia, the thalamus, and the cortex—networks that seemed intimately connected to helping the body move in an elegant and organized fashion.

Among the first investigators to come up with models of the basal ganglia's role in movement disorders was a team at the University of Michigan: Roger Albin, Ann Young, and Jack Penney . Their 1989 report, "The Functional Anatomy of Basal Ganglia Disorders," published in the journal *Trends in Neuroscience*, proposed that the movement problems stemming from these diseases resulted from changes in the activity of particular basal ganglia neurons, leading to an increase in basal ganglia output.[20] Abnormalities in these circuits would perturb movement and lead to all sorts of symptoms that appear not only in Parkinson's disease but also in dystonia and other movement disorders. DeLong's model, developed at Hopkins, was very similar; they all were on the right track. Understanding how these brain regions talked to one another, and what happened when the circuits were damaged, would lead to a generation of studies that turned the corner on the treatment of these disabling conditions.

For a while at least, the thalamus retained standing as a first-line target. By the late 1980s, Hopkins had recruited Canadian neurosurgeon Fred Lenz to develop a functional neurosurgery program, and his team—which included DeLong and Vitek—began doing thalamotomies for Parkinson's tremor. As neurologist-scientists, DeLong and Vitek were able to offer their expertise in the operating room to help locate brain regions. They would use microelectrode recording to listen to the language of different brain cells in order to guide the surgeons directly to where they needed to be in the thalamus. The patients were awake, so that doctors and the scientists could watch their behavior and gauge their physical and emotional reactions to avoid damaging key areas of the brain. Between surgeries, they worked in the laboratory to figure out how the thalamic cells were related to movement.

The functional organization of the motor regions of the thalamus—its characteristic physiological properties that would allow surgeons to identify the different regions when mapping with a microelectrode in the operating room—was unclear despite many efforts. Vitek and his colleague Jim Ashe began mapping the structure by performing multiple recording tracks through the region using the same electrode—a difficult feat. The results of this work, published in the *Journal of Neurophysiology*, helped the field to better understand how the thalamus was organized and shed light on the surgical targets in it.

By the time DeLong's *Science* paper on targeting the subthalamic nucleus in MPTP monkeys hit the presses in 1990, he had already accepted a post as chairman of the neurology department at Emory University in Atlanta. At Emory he decided to put together a movement disorders center. DeLong invited Vitek to help, and Vitek accepted. In order to start the center, DeLong and Vitek knew that they needed a neurosurgeon, and they didn't have to look far. Roy Bakay was a neurosurgeon at Emory. He had done a few thalamotomy procedures on Parkinson's patients, but it was when DeLong, Vitek, and Bakay formed a trio that surgery for movement disorders took off at Emory.

With bench science and animal experiments proving so informative and pallidotomy reemerging to relieve patients unable to benefit in the long term from L-dopa, it remained for researchers to produce one more series of advances that would open the road to deep brain stimulation. Those advances would emerge from the confluence of neurosurgery and revelations from microrecording of brain cells. They started to take shape when DeLong, Vitek, and Bakay began a series of studies of the neural circuits of these regions. These studies soon were followed by others, including those of a young neurosurgeon named Andres Lozano of the University of Toronto. In the 1990s, their reports on pallidotomy and physiology of the basal ganglia set the stage for a new generation of surgical treatments for movement disorders—and, in time, other neurological conditions. These studies would clarify the neural circuitry, refine the techniques for interrupting its abnormal activity, and settle, finally, on the globus pallidus as a key structure for surgery to relieve movement disorders.

Michael Dogali, a neurosurgeon at New York University, had been the first to take hold of Lauri Laitinen's idea and lesion the pallidum. DeLong, Vitek, and Bakay made a trip north to New York to watch him do the surgery in 1991, a year before Laitinen's paper was published. When they returned to Atlanta, Vitek began developing a system for Bakay's operating room so that they could do microelectrode recordings. If Vitek had learned anything from his years of recording from single cells in the laboratory, it was that patterns of spontaneous neural activity are different. And using microelectrodes that are no larger in diameter than a strand of hair can help surgeons identify exactly where they are in the brain. Vitek worked with Doug Real, who was in the Emory neurology department, and a postdoctoral fellow from Japan, Yoshiki Kaneoke, who was working in Vitek's primate laboratory. They set up the recording equipment for the Parkinson's surgeries by buying individual pieces and putting them together. The setup was similar to the one they were using in their animal facility.

Bakay, Vitek, and DeLong brought their first patient into the operating room on December 11, 1992. Steve Atchley, a Parkinson's patient in his thirties, was eager to be the first Emory patient to have the surgery. It began at eight in the morning, and they didn't finish until two o'clock the following morning—eighteen hours. "We didn't know whether the human basal ganglia would be organized in the same way as they were in the monkey," Vitek recalled in 2008. "We told him that we had never done a pallidotomy. He said he wanted to be the first."

The surgeons made a unilateral lesion on the right side of Atchley's brain. It was a success. His stiffness, slowness, and rigidity improved dramatically. Vitek remembers vividly that Atchley said he felt his arm start to relax at the very moment that the lesion was being made.

Waiting lists for the surgery swelled. At Emory, patients eventually faced a two-year wait for surgery—and that was on top of a two-year wait for an appointment just to get an evaluation for the procedure.

Meanwhile, Vitek, Bakay, and DeLong held off publishing the results until they had enough patients to see whether the lesioning surgery was working. And they wrote a federal grant to study the surgical procedure in a scientific way: comparing it with conventional medical therapy. (Patients who signed on and ended up on medical therapy for nine months were promised the surgery and received it within the study year.) In the end, their efforts paid off. They enrolled fifty-six patients and proved that the surgical lesion in the pallidum worked better than medications, reducing symptoms 30 percent more than the drugs. Many of the patients were followed over a two-year period, and the benefits of treatment persisted. The results of the study were published in the *Annals of Neurology* in 2003.[21]

The investigators moved away from the subthalamic nucleus (STN) with both reluctance and relief. The reluctance came from the STN's early emergence as a surgical target able to give dramatic improvement in the wake of DeLong and his colleagues' *Science* paper on the MPTP monkeys. A handful of neurosurgeons had done lesioning in the STN, and it was still an appealing target. At the International Center for Neurological Restoration in Cuba, neurosurgeon Julián Álvarez Blanco, neurologist José A. Obeso (from Spain), and their colleagues were testing the benefits of bilateral subthalamic lesions to treat Parkinson's on eighteen patients. Emory neurologist Jorge Juncos made several trips to the island and helped with the evaluation of the patients. The patients were followed for two years. At the end of the study, 50 percent of them still had significant benefit from the operation.

In the Cuban patients, the subthalamic surgery both diminished symptoms and helped reduce the L-dopa-induced dyskinesia—the wild, flailing dancelike moves—that afflicted patients after years on L-dopa. The study found two other notable benefits: patients were able to cut the doses of their medicines by 74 percent, and the surgery could be done relatively safely on both sides of the brain.

Many scientists were relieved to learn of subthalamotomy as an alternative, because they knew that bilateral pallidotomy could cause hypophonia, or quiet speech. Cognitive problems had also been associated with the surgery. Still, surgeons were leary of bilateral STN lesions because when the STN was damaged in humans, usually by a stroke, they developed hemiballismus, an involuntary movement disorder that consists of wild flinging movements. DeLong and Vitek had suggested trying an STN lesion, but even Bakay was hesitant, despite their work on monkeys that suggested hemiballismus did not occur in the Parkinson's disease state. Once Laitinen advocated globus pallidus lesions, this structure seemed a safer target.

With pallidotomy coming of age, STN was relegated to a backseat. Later, when deep brain stimulation, with its reversibility, emerged, it would allow scientists to step up to the STN and see what targeting it could do for patients.

Chapter 4

The French Connection

At age forty-five, Dr. Alim-Louis Benabid, an unassuming, creative, easygoing neurosurgeon at the University Hospital of Grenoble, France, became the father of high-frequency deep brain stimulation to quiet abnormally hyperactive regions of diseased brains. Neurologists and neurosurgeons had been looking for alternatives to the complete destruction of discrete brain tissue. Anywhere from 10 to 20 percent of patients had some side effects (at an even higher rate with surgery to both sides of the brain), and neither the surgery nor the problems that resulted were reversible. Benabid gave neurosurgeons something new and better for their patients. If stimulation didn't work, or if it did more harm than good, no problem; the device could be shut off and the battery pack removed.

Benabid had learned how to do experimental surgeries on animals in 1979 during a year-long postdoctoral fellowship in the laboratory of Dr. Floyd Bloom at the Salk Institute in La Jolla, California. At this premier research center, Benabid, who had just earned a doctorate in physics, began to listen to the electrical language of the brain. Active cells give off a static, hissing sound. If you listen long enough, you can hear the distinct language of specific cell types. "Floyd taught me that once you reach your target you have to stimulate at different frequencies because the results can be very different. Electrical stimulation is a means to excite the nervous system," said Benabid.

After his year in Bloom's preclinical neuropharmacology laboratory, Benabid headed back to his birthplace and resumed residency at Grenoble University—and he has never left. By the time Benabid was appointed head of the neurosurgery department of the University Hospital in 1989, surgery for Parkinson's disease, dystonia, and a small number of psychiatric conditions had already passed the test as acceptable treatment for worst-case patients who did not respond to available drugs. It was also becoming clear in the field of neuroscience that the brain works more like a battery than a soup of chemicals.

Benabid, like other neurosurgeons in the late 1980s, was doing ablative surgery—cutting, freezing, or burning precise brain tissue, a procedure saved for patients for whom all other therapies had failed. Benabid would send a small electrode into the area he wanted to lesion—usually the thalamus, to stop tremor—and stimulate the electrode at thirty to sixty hertz to make sure he was in the right place. If he got too close to the sensory thalamus, he could make the motor deficits worse and induce tingling on the opposite side of the body. He and his colleagues used low frequencies, which actually made the tremor temporarily worse, so they knew where they were heading.

In November 1986, Benabid's surgical team was operating on a man with essential tremor. They had threaded the electrode down into the thalamus and had started stimulating, climbing to one hundred hertz. Suddenly the patient's tremor stopped. "I was not prepared," Benabid recalled. "Initially, I thought I obtained a contraction because I was in the wrong place, in the internal capsule. I apologized to the patient."

"It's no problem," said the patient. "It was nice."

Benabid repeated the stimulation at one hundred hertz. The man moved his fingers, wiggling with the utmost control and surprise. The high-frequency stimulation had suppressed his tremor. Benabid continued with his original surgery to lesion an area of the thalamus called the ventral intermediate nucleus. He repeated the electrical stimulation on the next five patients. "I observed this phenomenon," Benabid explained. "At low frequency, the tremor would worsen. At high frequency, it would completely disappear." He thought that the high frequency was somehow mimicking the effects of a lesion.

Though neurosurgeons such as Irving Cooper in New York had implanted electrodes into the brain for the treatment of pain and movement disorders as early as the 1970s, these surgeons had missed the nuance of the procedure. The level of the frequency was one key to success. "In those early reports, you never even saw the word *frequency* written," said Benabid. "Nobody picked up on this important point."

Even Benabid had been using low-frequency deep brain stimulation in the thalamus to control phantom limb pain—a puzzling disorder in patients who have amputations and still perceive pain in the missing limb. His theory was that the electrodes would stimulate the sensory thalamus and trigger a perception of tingling that felt good to these patients.

"We had the method. We had the electrodes. We had the stimulating leads," Benabid said. "Why not try putting these electrodes into the same regions we were lesioning and stimulate with high frequency?" But even he needed convincing. There were no ethical committees to guide his way. He had a patient return to his office two years after a thalamic lesion had stopped tremors on one side of his body. Now the man was begging to have the other side done.

Benabid knew that bilateral lesions were complicated and risky. Patients who had bilateral surgeries tended to have problems talking and suffered from cognitive and memory deficits. Benabid was not willing to make life even worse for his patient.

"I have a proposition to make," he told the patient. "I believe we could do this with an electrode. And if it doesn't work, there is no risk. We'll just remove it."

Thus, in January 1987, electrodes were threaded into one side of the man's brain and were connected to a stimulating device. Benabid and neurologist Pierre Pollak kept increasing the frequency until the dial was set at one hundred hertz. "It was marvelous. The tremors stopped instantly," Benabid recalled. They closed the man's skull and left a cable dangling from his scalp. Every day they would return to his hospital room and stimulate the electrodes in his brain. And every day the tremors would stop. That same week, they tunneled the cable under the skin and through to a battery that was placed in his chest.

When the stimulator was on, no one could tell that this man had suffered for decades with a very severe resting tremor.

The neurosurgery to lesion key areas of the brain involved in movement disorders would now prove invaluable to teams of researchers who wanted to test the potential of deep brain stimulation. Surgeons had been putting electrodes into the brain during these procedures as a way to identify the terrain. The theory of the day was that stimulation inhibited neurons. It was Benabid's idea to leave the electrodes in place and to stimulate at high frequency that led to widespread testing of this new technique.[22] It was a radical idea, and no one knew what the long-term consequences would be. What happens when you insert electrodes into abnormal tissue and then send electricity into the tissue at a certain voltage, frequency, and amplitude?

By the time Mahlon DeLong's 1990 paper on the subthalamic nucleus was published, Benabid had implanted stimulating electrodes into the thalamus of dozens of patients, and they were happy with the results—at least for resting tremors. And Benabid also had been inspired by Laitinen to put electrodes into the globus pallidus in Parkinson's patients. By 1993, the French team had done around a hundred cases.

Thanks to DeLong's work, the subthalamic nucleus was a possible new target for Parkinson's, and Benabid was the first to test stimulation of the STN in patients. He began traveling to the United States to help push the technology forward. Benabid prepared very carefully for his approach to the STN. In the early 1990s, he made contact with Abdelhamid Benazzouz, a young scientist doing his postdoctoral thesis in Bordeaux. (Benazzouz is now a research director at Inserm, France's counterpart of the NIH.) Benazzouz had done deep brain stimulation in the STN in a monkey model, and he invited Benabid to sit in on the jury for his thesis. After Benabid had seen the results and had long discussions with Benazzouz, he was convinced that stimulation to this region would not cause dyskinesia, which was the main concern with lesioning. Benabid had been planning his own monkey study, but he abandoned it. Instead, he spent the next several months preparing the targeting, reading the anatomical literature, and comparing atlases of both human and monkey brains.

The subthalamic nucleus, unlike the globus pallidus, is small—a sliver of tissue harder to see on brain scans and more difficult to reach. Benabid actually saw this as an advantage. "While in STN, you are either in or out," he said. He scheduled his first patient for DBS-STN surgery on January 29, 1993. The procedure was done on only one side. A year later, the other side was done. In the interim, Benabid brought his second patient into surgery in July 1993, and both sides were done during one operation.

Benabid had already used Medtronic leads in six patients with tremor before he showed the company the results of his work. He presented the data and the videotapes of his patients before and after the procedure, and Mark Rise, a Medtronic engineer, and his colleagues were impressed. It came at just the right time. The company's engineers had developed a new electrode lead but had no application for testing it. The company had done some studies testing its usefulness to alleviate pain, but the effort was abandoned. Benabid's surgeries were proving that the stimulating electrodes could stop a clearly visible symptom—abnormal tremor—and that would make it a lot easier to sell to regulators in the United States than presenting a device that treated something as subjective as pain. "Changes in movement are pretty obvious," explained Rise, while "pain is something that is not so obvious."

Rise had a postdoctoral degree in engineering. He had joined Medtronic when the neurological division of the company was just taking off. The company had built its reputation on the first implantable heart pacemaker, and when Rise came aboard in 1980, pain theories that had emerged two decades earlier were making company scientists take a closer look at the electrical circuitry of the nervous system.

Rise arranged a dinner with Benabid at the 1993 annual meeting of the Society for Neuroscience. The French scientist agreed to help design the studies on the new electrode lead. The target for the international deep brain stimulation study was the thalamus. The condition they would treat was called essential tremor.

That same year, Benabid was invited to give a talk about high-frequency deep brain stimulation at a medical meeting in Ixtapa, Mexico. By this time, three years after reading DeLong's paper and another by a British group that also targeted the STN in two monkeys, Benabid already had put electrodes into the STNs of a few patients. He presented the preliminary results of these operations at the meeting. The target looked good so far.

At the meeting in Mexico, Todd Langevin, a vice president and general manager of global movement disorders for Medtronic, approached Benabid and asked an unusual favor. Langevin wanted Benabid to leave the sun and science in Mexico and fly to Florida to meet neurologist Warren Olanow and neurosurgeon Dr. Donald Smith, who were set to do their first DBS procedure on a patient with essential tremor. The target was the thalamus. Benabid agreed. When they arrived at the University of South Florida in Tampa, Benabid donned a pair of scrubs to join Smith and Olanow in the surgical suite. The patient on the table was George Shafer, who would appear before the 1997 FDA advisory panel hearing described at the beginning of this book.

DBS surgery was done while patients were awake and mildly sedated, so that the team could see quickly whether they were heading into risky terrain. The doctors had computerized maps of the target based on scans taken on Shafer the day before. They used these scans and maps to find their target and to thread the electrodes into the tissue. They passed thin electrodes into tissue along the way and stimulated them to listen to the sound of the neurons, which would guide them to the right tissue. When they reached their target, they put the electrode with four different contacts in place so that it could be stimulated and manipulated to find the best spot and frequency to calm the symptoms. When the first contact was turned on, Shafer's tremors stopped immediately. He asked for a piece of paper so that he could write his name. The words appeared on the page evenly. His hand was not shaking. Benabid recommended that they try another setting, which was common practice. But Shafer was so happy to see his hands quiet and steady that he said no, that would be all.

The next day, Benabid flew back to Mexico. A few months later, he received a picture of George Shafer building an intricate model airplane after his deep brain surgery.

By the mid-1990s, Medtronic had another study under way to test other brain targets for easing Parkinson's. DBS teams involved in the international trial would target either the internal segment of the globus pallidus (GPi) or the STN. Vitek and Bakay led the way at Emory, which was one of four U.S. centers enrolled in the study. DBS teams could pick either the GPi or the STN in each patient. Emory had four patients in the study. While the team felt more comfortable with GPi, since they had done extensive mapping of the region, they ventured out to place electrodes in the STN of two of their patients. Following completion of the study, scientists reported that there was a 30 to 50 percent improvement in symptoms, depending on the target and the programming. The results were published in the *New England Journal of Medicine*.

Benabid's studies using DBS for Parkinson's patients with advanced motor symptoms like rigidity and freezing would help Medtronic gain approval of the device throughout Europe. That was in 1998. Four years later, in 2002, a series of federal hearings was held to discuss the benefits and risks of the technique, and deep brain stimulation was approved for the treatment of Parkinson's in the United States.

It may sound as if all this was quick and easy, and as seismic changes in medicine go, the path to acceptance of deep brain stimulation—at least in the hands of neurosurgeons—was indeed fast. But to think that putting the procedure to work was as easy as, say, hooking up a DVD player would be a big mistake. Deep brain stimulation is a technique that goes beyond brain surgery. This is why it became clear right away to some of the people developing the technology that hospitals considering DBS would need teams of professionals—neurosurgeons, of course, but also neurologists, physiologists, psychiatrists, nurses, psychologists, and as they would come to learn, ethicists.

Medical professionals offering DBS had to figure out which patients were the best candidates. They needed to make each patient understand that DBS was an experimental procedure and that they could not promise success. Patients had to know the risks as well. As with any brain surgery, they could develop bleeding into the brain and die, become permanently impaired, or develop device-related infections. And there was a good possibility that their symptoms would not change once the electrodes were turned on at high frequency. But many patients who opted for the surgery lived with such disabling symptoms that they were willing to take the chance.

Patients would need presurgical MRI and CT scans so the team could map out the trajectory to their target. The information from the scans would be fed into a computer, and surgeons would use functional stereotactic techniques to identify where they needed to be. Patients had to be awake (and mildly sedated) to answer questions so that the team could ensure that they were not disturbing important brain regions on the way to their target.

Vitek and others also believed in using microelectrode recording to confirm the route and the final destination. Remember, each population of neurons has its own sounds, and listening to the sounds of the cells was critical if the surgeons wanted to hit the right spot. Not everyone thought that microelectrode recording was important, however. Some neurologists believed that the scans and the stereotactic programming could get them to the same place without risking further problems by threading hair-thin leads in and out of tissue to guide the course. The use of microelectrode recording is still debated in surgical halls today. No studies have been published comparing patients who had DBS with such surgical recordings to those who did not have the recordings. Yet Vitek said there is evidence that once the area is mapped with microelectrodes, surgeons often end up placing the lead in a location different from the one they originally targeted.

When the neurosurgeon arrived at the target, the team would guide a lead with four metal contacts into place. Having four contacts through which to stimulate expanded the possibility that if one contact did not diminish symptoms, another might. With the electrode in place, a programmer on the team would stimulate at each contact to gauge its effect. When they found the best response, they would turn off the stimulators, connect a wire to the lead, and send it out through the burr hole (the hole drilled through the skull) to finish part one of the surgery.

The next part of the procedure was to implant the battery in the chest wall and thread the lead—or leads if the procedure was done on both sides of the brain—down through the neck to connect the electrodes to a power supply. This was done under general anesthesia, often within a week of the surgery.

Programming was the final step in the procedure. Once a target was identified for stimulation, several steps were necessary to get the device working just right for each patient. The four contacts on the electrode were separated from each other by 0.5 or 1.5 millimeters. Stimulating through each contact led to a different effect. The idea was to find the contact that provided the most benefit with the fewest side effects and then to determine the best pulse width, frequency, and voltage. For Parkinson's disease, establishing a good setting for a patient could take three to six months because the disease brings a complex list of symptoms in addition to tremors. Each of several contacts required testing for every symptom, and all the other parameters were uniquely set to the patient's specific problems.

For tremor in patients who did not have Parkinson's, the procedure was relatively easy. Doctors knew they had the right contact and setting when the stimulation stopped a patient's tremor without side effects. The brain region that worked to alleviate tremor was the thalamus. Targeting the thalamus also worked for alleviating the tremor in Parkinson's disease, but these patients also suffered from other symptoms—rigidity, gait, and balance problems including freezing of the limbs—that did not respond to thalamic stimulation. And as the technique would be expanded to different diseases, including psychiatric conditions, and new tissue targets were identified and tested, it would become clear that offering DBS was a long-term commitment, on the part of both the DBS teams and the patients, who would have to figure out just how DBS was affecting their minds and bodies.

As the 1990s drew to a close, scientists continued to develop deep brain stimulation for movement disorders, and some began considering other uses for the technique. But a problem made it hard to frame hypotheses about its potential in other disorders: no one knew exactly how or why stimulating at high frequency worked. Boosting action in the cells seemed counterintuitive, considering the previous use of surgical cuts that destroyed the tissue permanently. Scientists speculated that stimulation acted like a lesion because it produced the same effects. But the best way to solve the riddle was for scientists like Vitek to study the basal ganglia circuits and related structures to figure out the mechanism behind the technique.

Vitek, then still at Emory, received funding from Medtronic to study the mechanism of deep brain stimulation. Just how did it work? This was a critical question that needed an answer. The study proposed placing stimulating electrodes into the subthalamic nucleus in an MPTP monkey with all the human features of Parkinson's. This would be one of a large number of studies on DBS that Vitek and his colleagues would do in the hope of helping the field find its way to new targets, new technology, and new applications. One of Vitek's postdoctoral fellows, Takao Hashimoto, took on the animal study with Vitek, while Vitek and Bakay were preparing the operating room for human patients.

Vitek had been bursting to develop a DBS program ever since reading the results of Benabid's work. Medtronic personnel, already thinking about other brain regions to target for the rest of the symptoms of Parkinson's, invited Vitek to become the principal investigator at Emory for a study on deep brain stimulation for the disease. The globus pallidus would be the target for the leads, but based on DeLong's work with MPTP monkeys, the Parkinson's study would also include stimulation of the subthalamic nucleus.

Vitek asked Bakay to join in the study, and Bakay agreed. But there was a vexing problem as they moved forward in the design. Remember that bilateral surgical lesioning of the thalamus and globus pallidus caused a host of disturbing symptoms that had kept surgeons away from destroying tissue on both sides of the brain. Instead, surgical teams chose the most severely affected side of the body in Parkinson's patients and operated on the opposite side in the brain. If, as speculated, stimulation mimicked lesioning, could they do it bilaterally without disabling side effects? It wasn't at all clear.

The new Emory team had taken their first patient, a woman with severe tremor, into surgery to implant electrodes into the thalamus in February 1997. As they began enrolling Parkinson's patients in the Medtronic-sponsored study, they started thinking about other conditions that might respond to deep brain stimulation of the circuitry they were investigating. Dystonia came to mind. Unlike Parkinson's, which causes slowed movement, rigidity, and tremor, dystonia causes muscles to contract involuntarily. The resulting spasms can run the gamut—from eye blinking to neck twisting to an entire body that seems bewitched. The mechanism that allows for the normal contraction and relaxation of muscles is off-kilter; the muscles don't get the message to relax. A patient with dystonia can contort into painful and awkward positions. Some patients with Parkinson's disease also develop dystonia.

Bakay and Vitek discussed the target for dystonia, for which lesioning was an established procedure. Because of the work that Cooper and others had done decades before, the thalamus was the selected target. When, in the summer of 1997, Bill Elkins arrived at their door seeking help, the discussion became concrete. Vitek and Bakay had operated on Elkins a year earlier, lesioning the GPi on one side. Now the dystonia patient was asking to have the other side done. They were reluctant to lesion the other side because they were concerned about the problems that had ruled out bilateral surgery of the globus pallidus for Parkinson's patients. However, Elkins's lesion surgery had given him only temporary relief from his dystonia. Vitek met with Elkins and his parents and decided that they would try deep brain stimulation on the other side of his brain.

When they were inside Elkins's brain, Vitek sent microelectrodes down to probe the region and to navigate his way to the GPi. He knew the language of the brain, its electrical sounds changing with each neuronal population. But he was heading through the GPi without realizing it, as it sounded like the GPe (the external segment), and it was only after he hit the optic tract that he realized he had gone through the GPi without knowing it. The experience was humbling. It was also a wake-up call indicating the importance of microelectrode recording to find the right target—or to know, in their case, that they had shot past it. At the same time, that the sounds of the cells of the two regions had not been different enough was an insight into the changes accompanying dystonia that would mean reevaluating the model of movement disorders based only on changes in the firing rates of cells.

Another event during this surgery would change the thinking about how deep brain stimulation worked in regulating abnormal brain circuits. When Vitek began programming the device, it had no immediate effect on Elkins's symptoms, unlike tremor or Parkinson's patients, who experienced relief from the stimulating electrode right away. They were all disappointed and thought that the technique just didn't work for the patient, or maybe even for the condition. Vitek was not sure what to do next. Should he give up or try to push the technology to see if it could help? He tried the latter. He turned up the parameters and told the programmer turning the dial that they would have to press on—even if they got a signal that tissue was at risk for damage from the high electrical current. His thinking was that if this didn't work, he could always go in and lesion the tissue, and he would have a ready-made target.

Elkins's symptoms remained unchanged the day after the initial programming, and the next day as well. Vitek discharged Elkins but asked that the family stay near for the weekend—just in case something happened, bad or good. That Sunday, Vitek got a call from the patient's mother: "Jerry, you won't believe it but Bill is standing straight." So the first case of deep brain stimulation for dystonia in the United States taught a lesson: the symptoms of dystonia are slow to respond, and it could take repeated programming to find the right settings for the abnormal movements to subside. On that Sunday, when his patient's body stood straight, Vitek recalled something that French neurologist Pierre Pollak had told him. Pollak's team had implanted stimulated leads into the brain of a dystonia patient, and when nothing happened they had removed the leads and sent a disappointed patient home.

Other teams bringing patients with dystonia into the operating room also noticed that the results were not immediate. In fact, it took a lot of programming and reprogramming of the device—finding the right lead, voltage, amplitude, and frequency—and it wasn't clear who would get better, or when.

"Nobody wanted to lesion if you could put stimulators in," Vitek recalled. And while neurosurgeons were moving toward deep brain stimulation, many questions were still unanswered. Should teams go after the GPi, a much bigger target, or the STN? Should electrodes be placed on one side or two? What's more, no one was collecting cognitive information on patients to see if the high-frequency stimulation was having any adverse effects on thinking, memory, or attention. Vitek was also concerned that some neurosurgeons were doing these procedures without using micro-electrode recording to help find the exact target.

To help answer some of these questions, Vitek, DeLong, and Bakay wrote another grant proposal and got funding to enroll 132 patients with Parkinson's disease. They randomly assigned the patients to either the GPi or the STN for stimulator implants on one side. They would follow these patients over time to figure out how many needed to have stimulators put into the other side of their brains, and to decide which target worked better. The team would also have the luxury of recording side effects and carrying out detailed neuropsychological and psychiatric monitoring. The study was funded in 1999, and it took more than eight years to enroll enough patients.

In May 2008, the study code (data on the patients and their responses, which is independently kept from the investigators so that they remain objective) was broken and the results were analyzed. Vitek had a month to prepare slides of the preliminary findings to present at a meeting in June. Although the data were still being organized and analyzed in June, the preliminary analysis that Vitek presented suggested that the overall effect using DBS in the GPi compared with the STN was not significantly different, based on a standardized scale (the UPDRS III motor score) used to assess the effect of DBS on the motor symptoms of Parkinson's. Vitek expected more detailed analysis of the results to reveal whether certain types of patients would do better with DBS at one site versus the other, whether one site or the other is more prone to side effects and what kind, or which patients would need DBS on a second side. That would provide scientists for the first time the data necessary to make a truly scientifically informed choice on whether one area—the globus pallidus or the subthalamic nucleus—would be better than the other. By then, virtually everyone in the DBS Parkinson's world was already implanting in the STN, following Benabid's direction. Vitek had thought that was a mistake, as only one small study with ten patients had compared the techniques over time, for Parkinson's or any other movement disorder. Vitek's current study had enough patients to be able to answer this question and also to determine whether patients would benefit from bilateral surgery.

For more than twenty years, since the mid-1980s, pioneering leadership—by DeLong, Laitinen, Benabid, and Vitek most notably—had been setting the landmarks by which deep brain stimulation could begin to advance. And so it did. A new generation of neurologists and neurosurgeons saw the technique's potential for solving some of the most vexing brain dilemmas—from intractable depression to snapping patients out of unconscious states.

Part Two

Tantalizing Leads

Chapter 5

Acting on Impulse
DBS and Dystonia

D eep brain stimulation began telling a story about the human brain, in health and in illness. Scientists were learning about the organization of the basal ganglia and figuring out how they could develop DBS for use in other brain problems, and deep brain stimulation was gaining momentum around the world. In New York, several teams were trying their hands with the electrodes. One of those surgeons was Ron Alterman. In 1994, Alterman was in a neurosurgery fellowship at the New York University School of Medicine, training under Dr. Patrick Kelly and Dr. Michael Dogali. Kelly, trained in France in classical stereotactic surgery, had become known worldwide for his work with brain tumors. When Alterman started his fellowship, Kelly was lesioning the thalamus for patients with tremor and Dogali had started a surgical program to lesion the globus pallidus.

Alterman had planned a one-year stay at NYU, but after Dogali left for the University of California at Irvine, he remained to work with Kelly, was given a faculty appointment in 1995, and continued at NYU until 1997, the same year the FDA approved deep brain stimulation for tremors. Alterman spent one year at the University of Pennsylvania doing thalamic stimulations before moving to New York's Beth Israel Medical Center as director of functional neurosurgery. Things were heating up in France, as Benabid was putting electrodes into the subthalamic nucleus. Alterman wrote the FDA asking for an investigational device exemption, or IDE, that allowed him to do the same thing—head into the subthalamic nucleus in patients with Parkinson's disease.

His first patient was a man in his forties with advanced Parkinson's. Alterman implanted electrodes on one side, planning to do the other side later. The symptoms on one side of the patient's body improved remarkably, but because he had postsurgical confusion, the second surgery was never performed. Alterman failed with his next patient. The sixty-eight-year-old had a hemorrhage and died. "We nicked the ventricular wall going in," said Alterman. "I have stayed clear of that wall ever since." Over time, the results of deep brain stimulation kept getting better and better, and there have been no more deaths from surgery at Alterman's hands.

In December 2000, Alterman received a phone call from Dr. Susan Bressman, a colleague at Beth Israel. Bressman was a movement disorder specialist who was part of a large team of scientists that identified and cloned the first gene for dystonia. She had a thirteen-year-old patient, a girl with a genetic mutation that triggered her movement disorder. Her body was in such crisis, thrashing around uncontrollably, that Bressman had to use medicines to put her into a deep sleep. "Can you put stimulators into her?" Bressman asked. While Vitek and Bakay at Emory and Andres Lozano in Toronto had already operated on patients with dystonia, Alterman's decision to help Bressman would alter the trajectory of his career. The young girl improved significantly with the stimulators in place, and Alterman and his colleagues began to see dystonia patients from all over the world.

About 300,000 Americans have dystonia. The condition can make patients twist, bend, and snap into postures that could rival those of any contortionist. Some lose control of the muscles in their neck, and others have limbs that move on their own, twisting their bodies into a pretzel on the floor. Dystonia is debilitating and painful. It is thought to be triggered in some cases by subtle genetic damage to the basal ganglia, the region that controls the coordination of body movements. Damage to the tissue causes electrical impulses between nerve cells and muscles to misfire, leading to contractions. Normally, muscles contract and relax, but in dystonia patients, muscles controlling opposing movements co-contract and lead to these abnormal and sometimes painful postures.

Alterman moved to Mount Sinai School of Medicine with neurologist Michele Tagliati to expand the DBS service and offer deep brain stimulation surgery to dystonia patients. They both had training with DBS from patients with tremor and Parkinson's. Alterman operated, and Tagliati was in charge of the adjustments of the pulse width, frequency, and voltage, as well as finding just the right place on the electrode tract to stimulate. For the most part, it was proving successful, but they were learning that it could take months of programming to find the right setting for each patient.

In 2004, Alterman and Tagliati were at a loss to help a man in his fifties with such severe dystonia that the entire trunk of his body would vault him into the air and down to the ground. Their target was the globus pallidus. The hope was to interrupt the pathway that was sending the abnormal signal from the brain to the muscles. Nine months after the stimulators were placed in his brain and turned on, the man was no better.

Then Tagliati decided to try a variation that had been looked at by Rajeev Kumar of Andres Lozano's group at the University of Toronto and more recently reported in a tiny study of three patients.[23] He reduced the frequency of the stimulator and used a deeper contact. (Remember that each lead has four contacts, and the multiple contacts allow doctors to hit different targets if one doesn't work.) Stimulating at high frequencies made the man's muscles pull and contract, so Tagliati reduced the frequency from 130 hertz to 80 and put a contact down closer to the sensorimotor region of the globus pallidus. Within a week, the patient's symptoms were virtually gone.

DBS for dystonia was also being done by Philippe Coubes and his colleagues at the Montpellier University Hospital in Montpellier, France. They had one of the largest collections of dystonia patients who had undergone DBS, but Alterman and his colleagues were catching up. By 2007, they had operated on seventy patients.

Tagliati began testing the benefits of lower-frequency deep brain stimulation in younger dystonia patients and found that it worked just as well as high-frequency stimulation. It also extended the battery power of the device, which was important because changing batteries meant another surgical procedure every two to five years.

One of their patients was captain of his school soccer team, whose foot had begun dragging at age thirteen. Tagliati diagnosed dystonia, and he was right. The boy tested positive for the DYT1 gene. The spasms were in the boy's knee. His parents had read about deep brain stimulation, and they wanted to put the electrodes in right away. So did the patient. Tagliati said no; it was not appropriate before trying any of the available medicines. In his heart, Tagliati knew it would do no good, but he had to try. Nine months went by without a change; the symptoms only grew worse.

A year after the diagnosis, the teenager braved the surgery, and eight weeks later he was playing soccer again. The Mount Sinai team completed a study of their youngest patients and found that they seemed to do better than adults. Tagliati no longer saw these kids as patients. They came back for annual checkups, and most were living without signs of the disease. But not everybody would do as well. Tagliati and Alterman knew that when they met a fifteen-year-old girl from Michigan named Madison.

Madison met all the developmental milestones of childhood; she walked and talked on schedule, and she learned to ride a bike. But when she entered the second grade, she began walking on the tips of her toes; her balance was off. And things grew worse, fast. She suffered such bad spasms that her body would curl around backward, her head touching the tips of her feet. Without warning, her body would close in on itself at her shoulder blades like a suitcase slamming shut. Her head would literally press against her backside.

Madison inherited the DYT1 gene from her mother, who also had dystonia, as did her own mother and two uncles. Madison's case was far more severe than her mother's. Her spasms took such a toll on her body that they consumed more calories than she could ever take in with food. At one point, she weighed in at thirty-nine pounds and was placed in hospice care, but she gained weight and returned home. One of her two brothers, three years younger, was following in her dystonic footsteps; he had to run instead of walk to keep his body balanced.

Diane Garchow, an aide at Madison's school, saw the family's chaotic home life and took in all three children. The two boys eventually returned to live with their mother, but Madison stayed with Garchow and her family. It would be hard to imagine a heart bigger or braver than Diane Garchow's; she had to constantly readjust Madison's body, and sometimes she was unable to unfold her and had to call an ambulance. "When she's stuck like that she has trouble breathing," said Garchow. Keeping weight on also continued to be a problem for Madison.

Michigan doctors placed stimulators in Madison's brain when she was eleven. For a short time, she was able to crawl and get dressed by herself. With physical therapy, she stood for the first time in years and could walk up to twenty feet before collapsing to the ground. An electrode became infected, and she had another operation to remove and replace it.

Excited by her renewed ability to stand and walk, Madison went to school and showed off her freedom. She fell. The fall sent her to the hospital, and again doctors put in a new set of electrodes because the first ones were no longer working. The new device offered no benefit to the girl, now a teenager. There were months when she couldn't even sit in her wheelchair because her spasms were so strong that she would break the headrest and the straps holding her in. That DBS offered little relief to Madison is not unusual, as you will see in future chapters that discuss the problems when deep brain stimulation is done without the proper training, teamwork, or follow-up.

Garchow, Madison, and Madison's brother went to a dystonia meeting in Chicago, where they met Alterman, who agreed to see Madison when he got back to New York. In December 2007, an organization called Wings of Mercy flew Madison and Garchow to New York twice, first for the surgery at Mount Sinai and then for the technical adjustments to get the settings just right. Alterman and Tagliati found a new lead setting that helped Madison slowly return to a world that she hadn't known in years. She wrote her homework by hand for the first time, and her muscles calmed enough to allow her to take in more calories than she burned while moving.

A month after the device was turned on, she weighed ninety pounds, and she could sit up and get up on all fours without help. She returned to school in March. "It's nice to be able to sit up and enjoy things around me," she said. "I love to be with my friends."

Even with the success of the new setting, to her doctors Madison was still a work in progress.

Some dystonia patients tried and failed so many treatments that by the time deep brain stimulation was on the table, it seemed like the brass ring. That was Robert Weil's story. As a child, he loved to listen to people's hearts through his father's stethoscope; he wanted to be an eye surgeon, just like his dad. In hindsight, little things in his childhood were clues to his future. His forehead would contract involuntarily, and his facial muscles seemed to have a life of their own. His handwriting was atrocious.

When Weil was in college, a bump on his forehead sent him to a doctor who noticed Weil's grimacing, constant eye blinking, and the wide lines on his forehead—evidence of either a lot of worry or a possible movement disorder. The physician suggested that Weil make an appointment with Dr. Howard Hurtig at the Graduate Hospital in Philadelphia. Weil's neck was now jerking in every direction. Hurtig diagnosed some kind of movement problem, likely dystonia, and gave him a prescription for Artane, a drug that dampened a chemical called acetylcholine and sometimes improved movement.

During the summer before medical school, Weil continually increased his Artane dose to try to control his movements, but the medicine didn't work. His vision was so blurry from the drug that it was as if the print of books and newspapers lifted off the page. He couldn't think straight.

When Weil started at New York University Medical School in August 1984, the Phi Beta Kappa student failed a test for the first time in his life. And then another and another. He was sent to the dean, who threatened him with expulsion if his grades didn't improve. The school sent Weil to a psychiatrist, Howard J. Kaplan, a luminary in his field. Kaplan put Weil through a battery of neuropsychiatric tests. He couldn't remember anything. He couldn't even pass a writing test that a kid in grade school would ace. Kaplan wondered how on earth the young man had gotten into medical school. Weil was afraid to tell him about the Artane because he thought he would be thrown out of medical school if they knew he had some kind of movement disorder. Kaplan referred him to another psychiatrist, Chaim Shatan, to whom he finally confessed the Artane. "That explains everything," the doctor said. "You have severe anticholinergic toxicity from too much Artane. It's amazing you even remember your name."

Another doctor diagnosed Weil with Tourette syndrome, a condition best known for its victims blurting out obscenities, though that is not a major symptom for most patients. More common symptoms are uncontrollable, repetitive movements. This doctor handed Weil a prescription for Haldol, an antipsychotic drug then widely prescribed for schizophrenia but also used for Tourette. Weil took one dose of Haldol and found himself in class with his body completely out of control, a severe reaction known as akisthesia. He wanted to jump out of his skin. Weil got out of the classroom, knocking over things in his path, and flushed the rest of the pills down the toilet.

Shatan referred Weil to Oliver Sacks, the British-born neurologist and author of two best-selling books, *Awakenings* and *The Man Who Mistook His Wife for a Hat, and Other Clinical Tales.* Sacks was well versed in movement disorders, and when Weil arrived at the doctor's small house in a waterside community just east of the Bronx, Sacks took one look at him and said simply but with abundant warmth, "You have dystonia." Along with the diagnosis, Sacks gave him a signed copy of *The Man Who Mistook His Wife for a Hat.* "How much do I owe you?" the medical student asked. Sacks stared blankly. "I don't know. How much do consultants make?" Weil took out fifty dollars in cash, put it on a table, grabbed his signed book, and left.

In his new land called dystonia, Weil learned that the condition was caused by a genetic mutation. By then his parents had divorced and his father was about to remarry. He took the wedding as an opportunity to play doctor and drew blood from ten of his father's family members. And before his father took his vows for the second time, Weil pulled him into an anteroom overlooking a New Jersey lake and asked him to roll up his sleeve. The vials of blood were sent to a laboratory in Florida for genetic testing. It was concluded that Weil had inherited the disease from his father.

In 1988, botulinum toxin type A, famous now as Botox, was an experimental medicine, but Weil was willing to try anything—even a medicine developed from the toxin that caused botulism. Botox could relax muscles, which for many patients helped calm their abnormal movements, including some forms of dystonia. The needle used to deliver the toxin was about two inches long and was directed into Weil's forehead and, later, his neck. Each treatment involved sticking the needle into his neck about twenty times to deliver four hundred Botox units—compared with the less-than-twenty-five-unit dose now routine for reducing wrinkles. It worked somewhat, but not enough.

In 1990, Dr. Paul Greene admitted Weil to Columbia Presbyterian Hospital to evaluate a potential treatment for his dystonia. It involved injecting baclofen, an antispasm medicine, between the bones of his spine into the fluid that bathes the brain. If this worked, he could have a baclofen pump installed. The first day brought no change, nor the second, and Dr. Greene decided not to try it a final time. The young man viewed this as his last chance at a normal life. That night, though his hospital room was less than a mile from the George Washington Bridge, a dense fog over Manhattan prevented Weil from seeing the massive structure on the skyline. To Weil, it was a metaphor for his life; he cried himself to sleep and, for the first time in his life, thought seriously about suicide.

By 1991, Rob Weil's contractions were so severe that they broke the small bones on his vertebrae (called pedicles) attached to his neck muscles, and his back had curved so much from the irregular muscle contractions that his height had been reduced by an inch. The Botox was no longer working—the human body develops antibodies to the toxin and it loses its power. The medicine was also too expensive, at almost five thousand dollars for each treatment.

Weil had graduated from medical school in 1988 and was married with two young children. Taking care of his patients was getting more and more uncomfortable. He looked sicker than they did. "In rounds, I would lean up against a wall and press the back of my head firmly against the wall so I could keep my neck from pulling backward," he recalled. "It was painful." His marriage dissolved in 1995.

In 1999, some surgeons were ablating select peripheral nerves to treat dystonia. Weil was evaluated for the procedure at Beth Israel Medical Center, but his symptoms were so widespread across his back that he wasn't a candidate. While there, however, he met neurosurgeon Ron Alterman, who had placed electrodes in hundreds of Parkinson's patients with success and already had done so for five patients with dystonia. "You need it," the neurosurgeon said after a brief exam and a review of Weil's chart. The surgery would cost about $100,000 and probably would not be covered by insurance, as the treatment was not yet approved by the FDA. But Weil was ready to do anything to live a normal life, to practice medicine without scaring his patients off, and to read to his kids without having to lie down with his head flat against a mattress. He would sign on to the surgery no matter what.

The surgery took six hours, with Weil awake so the team could evaluate his brain function during electrode placement. As is the standard for brain surgery, his head was bolted to the table with four screws drilled into his skull so it could not move even a millimeter. With Parkinson's, DBS surgeons guide the electrodes to the target in the brain and turn on the stimulation. They either hit the right spot or not. If not, they move the electrode until the patient's body stops its abnormal movement. Dystonia, for unknown reasons, is different. The target was the globus pallidus, but stimulating the region during surgery didn't inform them whether it would work.

For months after the surgery, Weil traveled from his home in Hershey, Pennsylvania, to Manhattan every two weeks for adjustment of the device. Doctors would reprogram the settings on the battery and increase the voltage. During these adjustments, sometimes his face would droop or his tongue would twist around in his mouth. Sometimes he became short of breath or couldn't speak. Finally, the DBS team got to the point where they found the right settings to almost eliminate his neck spasms without any of these side effects.

Weil's euphoria lasted only a few weeks; the spasms returned. After another round of trips to Manhattan to get the device working again, he wanted it out. But Michele Tagliati, his neurologist at Beth Israel, urged him to give it more time. Soon, his neck was not turning as vigorously as it had; it was beginning to work, after all. Then it stopped. This roller-coaster effect took him back to Manhattan again.

A diagnostic test of the DBS device showed it was not working. Tagliati stimulated each of the four contacts on the lead. Nothing. It turned out that two leads had broken; the wires threaded under his skin from the brain electrodes through the neck and down into the chest to the batteries were not strong enough to endure the constant spasms in his neck, whose arching movements were powerful enough to break bones—and, apparently, electrical wires. Alterman tunneled under Weil's scalp to replace the broken leads.

After the wire replacement operation, the electrodes deep inside Weil's brain were turned back on and, after two years of adjustments, the settings were nearly perfect. Robert Weil became a doctor who didn't need a wall to hold up his head and a father who could run and bike with his children, now teenagers. He ultimately fell in love and remarried.

In April 2003, the FDA gave permission for DBS teams to operate on patients with dystonia under a humanitarian device exemption. No studies were required by the government agency, because dystonia is a rare disease and the technique seemed to work. But scientists are studying patients with dystonia to see how effective DBS is. About two hundred people have had stimulators implanted for dystonia. In one study, twenty-two patients have been followed for three years, and scientists report that their disability scores have improved by about 50 percent. Not all patients respond to the treatment, but even modest improvements can help with the quality-of-life issues that so many people with dystonia face every day.

Chapter 6

Obsessive-Compulsive Disorder
DBS for Psychiatry

People marvel at the concept of deep brain stimulation when they see someone with advanced Parkinson's who is no longer jerking and can walk smoothly, or a young boy out playing basketball again after being unable even to sit in a wheelchair without falling to the ground because of dystonia. But then mention that neurosurgeons and neurologists have teamed up with psychiatrists to tackle obsessive-compulsive disorder, Tourette syndrome, or depression, and there is a look of consternation. Stimulating the brain to alter behavior and mood? It harkens back to the unfortunate history of psychosurgery, in which doctors removed frontal lobe tissue from patients with all sorts of psychiatric diseases in the name of altering bizarre behavior and thinking.

And yet the modern-day pioneers in deep brain stimulation learned from working with patients with movement disorders that a turn of the stimulation dial could create changes in mood and behavior. Such side effects had been noticed early enough that well designed studies such as those by Vitek and Andres Lozano at the University of Toronto had routinely included gathering data on changes in mental status as part of measuring outcomes in patients treated with DBS for movement disorders.

However, invasive procedures for psychiatric conditions have always fallen under the shadow of the lobotomist Walter Freeman. Beginning in the 1930s, Freeman, a neurologist and psychiatrist with no surgical training, went around the United States sticking an ice pick through patients' eye sockets into the frontal lobe in an attempt to treat psychiatric conditions like schizophrenia. He performed about 3,500 such procedures, which he called transorbital lobotomies, in almost half the states in the country. Freeman conducted some of these lobotomies with neurosurgeon James Watts, who eventually broke relations with him. Freeman continued performing lobotomies on his own. His most famous patient was Rosemary Kennedy, who was rendered incapacitated after he took swipes at her frontal cortex. She was twenty-three. (For a complete history of psychosurgery, read Jack El-Hai's *The Lobotomist*.[24])

Lobotomies almost completely stopped when the first antipsychotic drugs came along in the 1950s. But for many severely ill patients, the medicines either didn't work or left them with terrible side effects. Scientists who were studying the brain began to refine surgical procedures to help the most intractable patients find some relief from their symptoms.

With modern techniques in hand, surgeons in the 1980s and 1990s quietly returned to the operating room with their worst psychiatric cases. Unlike their neurosurgical predecessors, they had brain scans and computer maps, tools that this new generation of psychiatrists hoped would help them identify areas involved with depression and obsessive-compulsive disorder (OCD). These surgeries were not as dangerous as in the past, and many patients awoke with their symptoms gone or at least greatly diminished.

In the 1990s, lesioning the cingulate—one of the brain's emotional, or limbic, structures—was resurfacing as a surgical option for people with intractable obsessive-compulsive disorder. The procedure involved piercing the cingulate with a long, thin electrode. Since it was first introduced in the 1960s, about a hundred patients had undergone it. In 1991, in the *Archives of General Psychiatry*, Michael Jenike, associate research chief of the Massachusetts General Hospital department of psychiatry, and his colleagues reported on thirty-three patients who had undergone the procedure for OCD since the mid-1960s. Employing a combination of questionnaires and telephone interviews, they concluded that the symptoms of 25 to 30 percent of the patients were substantially reduced even decades after surgery.[25]

The journey toward deep brain stimulation for OCD began in earnest in 1994, when Steven Rasmussen, a psychiatrist at Butler Hospital (an affiliate of Brown University), teamed up with colleagues at the Karolinska Institute in Sweden to perform gamma knife radiosurgery in patients with severe cases of OCD. In this surgery, no incisions are made. Instead, surgeons target the abnormal tissue—in this case the anterior limb of the internal capsule—and aim radiation beams at the target. Because each radiation beam is too weak to harm normal tissue, it does damage only to the area surgeons want to target.

The limbic structures of the brain modulate mood and behavior. As far back as 1949, a French neurosurgeon, Jean Talairach, had introduced a lesion to the anterior limb of the internal capsule, a small region connected to fronto-thalamic pathways. Lars Leksell also performed a number of these procedures and developed the technique well into the 1950s, and Ernest Spiegel and Henry Wycis reported that dorsomedial thalamotomies improved OCD symptoms. Whether patients really got better was anyone's guess. It was hard to interpret: case reports suggested that 25 percent of patients improved somewhat and an equal number got worse. But these patients were suffering despite the medications they swallowed, and surgery was seen as a hopeful option for their desperate situations.

The scientists at the Karolinska Institute went back into the charts of patients operated on two decades earlier and found that those who had gotten well had something in common: the surgeons had damaged the intended target, the anterior limb of the internal capsule. Those who were off their mark had patients who didn't get better, and some even got worse. Many surgeons used the gamma knife and thermal lesions to damage the tissue. The surgery is still done today, and doctors at the Karolinska Institute, Brown, and Harvard are conducting a placebo-controlled study to test the benefits of gamma knife capsulotomy.

These surgical lesioning experiences did have a benefit, however. Because destroying this tissue worked for some OCD patients, researchers figured the target had some potential when testing deep brain stimulation.

Bart Nuttin, a professor of neurosurgery at the Katholieke Universiteit Leuven in Belgium and head of the clinic of neurosurgery in the University Hospitals Leuven, was the first surgeon to consider placing stimulating electrodes in a patient with obsessive-compulsive disorder. In 1998, he had placed electrodes into the anterior limb of the internal capsule in two patients but had not seen a clear benefit.

Nuttin worked with two psychiatrists, Loes Gabriels and Paul Cosyns, and they continued to bring OCD patients into their operating suites. Rasmussen, an expert on obsessive-compulsive disorder, was introduced to Nuttin by Medtronic's Mark Rise. Nuttin invited Rasmussen to Belgium just in time for his second surgery in 1999. Also in the operating room that day was Bjorn Myereson, from the Karolinska Institute. Nuttin and his colleagues saw some success with their next few patients.

Nuttin's initial observations meant that deep brain stimulation could possibly take the place of damaging even small amounts of tissue. Not surprisingly, his target was the anterior limb of the internal capsule tissue. Located between the caudate and the putamen that interconnects large regions of the frontal lobes involved in mood and anxiety, this tissue hooks up into a network of interconnected regions that together regulate human mood, anxiety, and behavior. Nuttin saw the internal capsule as a major hub of the brain, connecting various critical areas on the surface of the brain to the deeper limbic regions. All the roads converge along the fiber tracts of the internal capsule like trains coming in and out of New York's Grand Central Station. The internal capsule is the track along which the trains operate.

Back in the United States in 2000, Rasmussen called on Benjamin Greenberg for help in his studies of the benefits of gamma knife capsulotomy. A psychiatrist at the National Institute on Mental Health working on transcranial magnetic stimulation for the treatment of depression, Greenberg was also a master imager. Rasmussen and Greenberg's plan was to take snapshots of the brain in OCD patients undergoing the surgery to make a small lesion in the internal capsule.

The first patient they brought to the federal campus in Bethesda was a young woman with such bad OCD that she couldn't go through a doorway when anyone else was nearby. With a busy NIH clinical center and a large set of double doors, it took Greenberg and Rasmussen an hour to get her up to the scanning machine. Then she was asked to take her jewelry off because of the high magnetic fields in the scanner. That was impossible, the woman said. She could take her jewelry off only in the upstairs bathroom of her Long Island home. Greenberg carefully cut out little paper models that he used as tubes over the patient's fingers and safely removed the jewelry without causing her undue anxiety.

Greenberg became fascinated by obsessive-compulsive disorder. In 2000, Rasmussen recruited him to Brown University and Butler Hospital in Rhode Island to head deep brain stimulation studies, first in obsessive-compulsive disorder and then, three years later, in depression. Greenberg extended the collaboration to include neurosurgeon Ali Rezai, psychiatrist Donald Malone, and others at Cleveland Clinic who wanted to move the technique beyond movement disorders and intractable pain. This group of doctors understood that only an interdisciplinary team of specialists working together can set up the optimal scenario: the most comprehensive and accurate patient selection, surgical procedure, postoperative management, and outcome and complication assessments. In 2002 the University of Florida group would join them, and these three U.S. medical centers would begin a study that would test the benefits of DBS for psychiatric diseases. But that was still to come.

The Brown and Cleveland team received federal and local approval to operate on ten of their most difficult patients. The pilot study was funded by Medtronic. The Brown group implanted deep brain stimulators in their first OCD patient in 2000.

After the stimulators were turned on and painstakingly set and reset over the long-term follow-up, about half of these severely disabled and medication-intractable patients responded to DBS, as defined by more than 35 percent improvement on standardized scales such as the Yale-Brown Obsessive Compulsive Scale (Y-BOCS).

In 2001, Rasmussen, Greenberg, Rezai, and Malone flew to Belgium to meet with Bart Nuttin. After the first few cases, Nuttin, Rasmussen, and Greenberg reviewed patient outcomes. They thought they had identified a better target where the fibers connected the thalamus to the medial and orbital cortex that ran through the capsule. It was lower down in the brain than the classic "Grand Central Station" target. And it proved to work.

In the operating room, they began going deeper into the brain and narrowing their target to a network of fibers connecting the anterior capsule, the anterior commissure, and the posterior ventral striatum. By 2008, 60 percent of their patients were getting better—not *all* better, but well enough to fall in love, to get work, to raise kids, and to spend far more time without symptoms than with them. But deep brain stimulation for psychiatric conditions was very much a work in progress. These experiments called for careful patient selection, study, and follow-up to figure out the short- and long-term benefits and risks of putting electrodes into the brains of patients who were often so disabled that they couldn't function normally. And these were the patients who were resistant to virtually every medicine they were given.

OCD affects about 1 to 3 percent of the U.S. population—between five million and eight million Americans. The disorder can take several forms, which translate into types. "Ritualizers," for example, are forever washing their hands or showering for fear of contamination. "Checkers" constantly doubt their actions and spend inordinate amounts of time backtracking and making sure appliances or lights are off. And "hoarders" compulsively hide objects, even some with no apparent value. For many, OCD begins in childhood. About 20 percent of patients fail to respond to traditional therapies, medicine, or behavioral techniques.

Mario Della Grotta of Providence, Rhode Island, had such severe OCD that he had no time for a normal life. He woke up at four thirty in the morning and started counting, checking, arranging, and cleaning. Numbers consumed him. He had more than two thousand telephone numbers stored in his head, and every day provided the opportunity for even more to memorize. This counting ritual had begun in childhood; books, clothes, underwear—anything that came in a quantity greater than one—provided a source of obsession. As a child he wrote his name thousands of times, on any kind of surface, including his legs. He made art out of his own name before moving on to signatures of famous people. Papers had to line up just right. As he got older, he spent countless hours on making calculations, figuring out bills, arguing with waitresses about a difference of a few pennies, and memorizing entire chapters from college textbooks.

The problems became more severe when Della Grotta became a young adult. After he married, his wife, Sheri, noticed that the spices in the drawer were lined up in alphabetical order. The cabinets were grouped by foods and the sizes of the jars and cans. One day, she went into the junk drawer and messed things up. Mario cried. "I think you have obsessive-compulsive disorder," she told her husband. Sheri worked at Butler Hospital, and she urged him to get help.

The first doctor he saw sent him over the edge. The OCD expert kept Della Grotta waiting for thirty minutes, and when he walked into her office there were papers stacked, rather unevenly, everywhere. He tried one medicine after another, and nothing broke his daily cycle. He was sent to McLean Hospital's inpatient OCD program in Belmont, Massachusetts. The staff wouldn't let him shower, at least not the way he was accustomed to: long and frequent rituals that took a few hours every day. His stay was short-lived. He walked out and found his way back to Rhode Island.

Della Grotta's early-morning rituals exhausted him. Brush teeth, shower, brush teeth, shower, shower, brush teeth, shave, shower. Finally, he moved into the closet and counted the ties and the shoes and the pants; then he was on to the kitchen, with so many things to count and arrange and rearrange. Money took up a lot of space in his rituals. By 9 a.m. he would go over the bills, accounting for every penny.

One night, on the way home from a bachelor party, he retraced every last cent of the hundred dollars he had had with him. He got to ninety-five dollars, as he made a mental image of what he had used the money for. But where was the remaining five? He pulled over on the side of the road, and numbers crammed his brain. He spent four hours ruminating about the night and the missing money, until a state trooper on his second round that evening pulled up and asked if he was all right.

"I'm stuck," Della Grotta said. While his car was running fine, his mind wasn't. The state trooper made him drive home. It was 4 a.m. Twenty minutes later he realized that he had spent the five dollars on a raffle ticket.

By the time Della Grotta met psychiatrist Benjamin Greenberg at Butler Hospital, every treatment had failed him. Greenberg was just gearing up for the experimental study on deep brain stimulation, and Della Grotta wanted in; he was about to become a father for the first time. Greenberg wanted Della Grotta to try another round of medicines before being accepted into the study. Della Grotta wasn't at all happy about it, but he did it. He didn't get any better.

In February 2001, Della Grotta settled into the halo that would hold his head down for the lengthy procedure and watched as Rasmussen, Nuttin, Greenberg, and Butler neurosurgeon Gerhard Friehs took their places at the surgical table and began operating on his brain. He was the first American patient in the international study.

No one could promise that it would work. DBS had not been a home run for OCD, but even a base hit would be acceptable. On the operating table, with the electrodes in place and turned on, Greenberg attempted to worsen the anxiety of his patient by dropping coins into his hand. Della Grotta's anxiety scorched the air. The stimulator was turned on, and he reported that the pennies were not bothering him as much. The surgeons turned the knob up, sending more electricity to the electrodes until Della Grotta's anxiety levels fell to normal. They had arrived at the spot that they believed would relieve many of his symptoms. When the stimulator was turned off, Della Grotta immediately dropped the coins from his hand. No one really knew how things would play out for a patient like this once he left the hospital.

Following the surgery, Della Grotta agreed to continue taking medicines and doing behavior therapy with hopes that all the treatments would work together. It would take many months before his symptoms diminished enough for him to live most of his day without checking or counting or rearranging his world. The symptomatic behaviors were down to four hours instead of fourteen.

In May 2005, Della Grotta received his BS in paralegal studies from Johnson and Wales University in Providence. His psychiatrist and psychologist advised him to study like a C student, and he did. No longer did he memorize pages of textbooks; he read his notes the night before an exam rather than weeks beforehand; and he walked out with a 3.23 GPA.

The DBS device altered Della Grotta's life in dramatic ways, but he, his wife, and his team of doctors and therapists learned to be mindful of its pitfalls. One day, Della Grotta, a diabetic, was not feeling well, and Sheri urged him to drive to the emergency room. On his way, another state trooper entered his life. This time Della Grotta was pulled over.

"I'm diabetic and driving to the hospital," he told the trooper. "I'll call an ambulance, just stand by," the trooper said. "Then I'll call a tow truck to take your car home."

Della Grotta still couldn't deal with germs, and just the thought of a germ-laden ambulance made him panic. He declined the trooper's offer, rolled up his car window, and began counting and counting. His OCD symptoms were back with a vengeance, and he had no idea why.

The ambulance arrived, and so did the tow truck. Everyone outside was banging on Della Grotta's window as he sat there stunned and counting, unable to unlock himself from the car or the situation. When he saw the trooper heading back to his car, Della Grotta took off. The ensuing chase ended when the trooper broke the driver's-side window and physically removed Della Grotta from the car. By the time he arrived at the hospital, by ambulance and now in handcuffs, Benjamin Greenberg was there to give the trooper a short course on OCD. Later that evening, Greenberg tested Della Grotta's device, and the battery was on its way out—hence the exaggerated symptoms. The same month, Della Grotta was brought back to surgery and was given a new battery and a way back to a more normal life.

In the United States, the government was handing out its first grants for other studies to test DBS for obsessive-compulsive disorder. The first approved grant went to psychiatrist Wayne Goodman at the University of Florida in Gainesville. Greenberg worked with the Florida group to develop their program. They brought half a dozen OCD patients into surgery. (Goodman is now at the National Institutes of Health.)

However eager American psychiatrists were when studying the results of European studies and starting to craft their own, they were interested in more than just results. Selling psychiatric neurosurgery in America—even a reversible procedure like deep brain stimulation—would have to proceed carefully and with respect to the abuses of the past. Ethics had been a concern from the beginning.

Stimulation offered opportunities for a wider audience than ablation surgeries, which are still being done for obsessive-compulsive disorder today. The fact that DBS worked to reduce symptoms in many patients failed by every other treatment opened the door to other vexing psychiatric conditions. But it also got them thinking and talking about the ethical dilemmas at hand: Who were the right patients? What were the right targets in the brain? What could they promise patients? And how could they avoid repeating the horrors of past surgical abuses against psychiatric patients?

As early as 2000, when Greenberg and Rasmussen started making plans, they put together an independent review committee of psychiatrists, ethicists, community members, and a professional informed-consent monitor. The consent monitor's job was to ensure that patients understood that DBS was an experimental technique and that there were no guarantees it would work. The consent monitor was David Shire, a chaplain who had done behavior therapy with patients who had religion-based obsessive-compulsive disorder. The team also called upon a physician-bioethicist at New York's Weill Cornell Medical Center, Joseph Fins, who agreed that the time was right to try DBS for the small group of psychiatric patients for whom all other forms of treatment were failing. Fins developed an ethics statement, which centered on the importance of psychiatrists treading carefully as they select and monitor DBS patients.

In France, the father of DBS, Benabid, was eyeing the work of his Belgian colleague, Bart Nuttin, and the American teams using deep brain stimulation for OCD. He was thinking about implications, too. In January 2002, Benabid invited scientists to meet in Aix-les-Bains, France. He was intrigued by the idea of treating psychiatric conditions with deep brain stimulation, but he was afraid of the legacy of the Freeman era of psycho-surgery. He invited Fins to talk about the ethics of the surgical treatment.

Fins, who was already steeped in the issues of using DBS for patients who may not have the cognitive abilities to make an informed decision, had entered bioethics by way of the palliative-care world. He had developed a way of thinking about affirming the right to care for terminally ill patients and at the same time preserving the right to die. He knew that helping to create guidelines for psychiatric conditions, in this case obsessive-compulsive disorder, would help lay the foundation for his next bioethics venture: a study using deep brain stimulation to reawaken brain regions of people in minimally conscious states.

What Fins had learned from working with dying patients was that they have to find meaning in a narrow window of time. What he learned from working with brain-damaged patients was that they have to rediscover who they are in the present and come to terms with what they lost, as well as the expectation of what could have been. He began to think about and address a neuro-palliative ethic of care founded on this common search for meaning and the need to balance the right to die with the right to ongoing care. With psychiatric patients, he had to be sure that they were ethically protected against any abuse, and that they understood what the technique was and that it was still experimental and potentially of no use. He was also keenly aware of the importance of getting the ethics right, given the dark legacy of psychosurgery, a topic often linked to the discussions of DBS in psychiatry.

By 2002, when he was addressing Benabid's scientific guests (investigators and clinicians), Fins had already created the ethical framework for the DBS study with minimally conscious patients. And he was happy to turn his attention to obsessive-compulsive disorder and ultimately to serve as senior author of the group charged with writing ethical guidelines for DBS in psychiatric disorders. Fins thought that the Aix-les-Bains gathering was remarkable. He was impressed with Benabid's willingness to tackle the ethical issues and to invite Didier Sicard, president of France's National Consultative Bioethics Committee, to be part of the discussion.

After the meeting, French neurosurgeons received permission to conduct a trial on DBS for OCD, and later that year the ethical guidelines were published. The list of guidelines consisted of nine points. It called for an ethics committee to work on all DBS studies and to evaluate each patient to ensure that every candidate meets certain medical and psychiatric criteria. It said the consent process should be tightly monitored. And while the candidates should have severe and chronic symptoms that have not responded to current therapies, DBS should be limited to patients who have the cognitive ability to make decisions based on a clear understanding of the procedure and its potential benefits and risks. The use of DBS in psychiatric patients should occur only at clinical research centers that can offer regular psychiatric follow-up visits, and a team approach, with neurosurgeons and neurologists working with psychiatrists and psychologists, should be mandatory. Also, investigators must disclose potential conflicts of interest to regulatory bodies and ethics committees. An important ethical guideline for psychiatric treatment is that the surgery should be performed only to restore normal function and to relieve patients' distress and suffering. And finally, no psychiatric surgery should ever be done for political, legal, or social purposes.

Marwan Hariz, a neurosurgeon at the University Hospital in London, said that the committee should have made a tenth guideline. He thinks that all patients enrolled in any DBS trial for mental illness should be followed and accounted for. He said that two of Nuttin's first patients, who did not respond to DBS, had been left out of his first paper when it was published in *The Lancet* in October 1999. Hariz, who studied under Laitinen, said that it is as important to talk about failures as it is to discuss successes.

By 2008, the collaborative international team had prepared a manuscript of the results of twenty-six patients with obsessive-compulsive disorder. One woman with breast cancer died a year after DBS implantation and was not included in the analysis. Stimulation was stopped in three patients who did not improve enough after a year of treatment to warrant keeping the device in. A fourth patient had the device removed, and when his symptoms continued to worsen he was taken into surgery for a capsulotomy three years after the study was completed.

The team used a series of behavioral rating scales to figure out whether or not patients improved with stimulation. At the end of the study, almost three-quarters of the patients had improved—their symptoms reduced but not completely eliminated. About 65 percent of the group was rated as "much better," and none were shown to be worse as a result of the treatment.

Now a new idea was stirring. In 2006, at an international neurosurgical meeting, the life of Mario Della Grotta, the Brown University team's early patient, was condensed into a few impressive slides presented by Ali Rezai of Cleveland Clinic. It was part of a talk on DBS for OCD that included eight other patients, each with his own story and measure of success. All had had electrodes placed bilaterally in the ventral capsule/ventral striatum (VC/VS) region, and after two years the scientists felt the procedure was safe and effective for those, like Della Grotta, who had tried everything else. Another patient, a nun who had spent her days checking for signs of contamination, found that the electrodes freed her from her fears. She began socializing more with the nuns who had taken care of her for decades.

Della Grotta, the nun, and others with OCD had started Greenberg and his colleagues considering the idea that DBS might help people with depression. In all the OCD patients who had been treated with DBS, a concomitant improvement in mood had been noted. This led the group to design a new clinical trial of DBS for depression. "The first thing we saw was changes in mood," Rezai said. "With the stimulator turned on, the nun's vision grew clear and she felt, like the others, that the weight of the world had lifted." Unfortunately, the nun had undiagnosed breast cancer at the time, and she died not long afterward. The doctors were given permission to study her brain to further their research, and now they had proof that the stimulators had reached their target with no damaging effects to the tissue.

Chapter 7

DBS Teams
Take On Depression

Surgery for depression was not new. In the lobotomies of the 1940s, surgeons saw benefits, but they also knew they had to search for ways to prevent the disastrous effects of swiping at large regions of brain tissue. They began targeting connections between prefrontal structures and deeper brain areas such as the thalamus and the basal ganglia. Such operations continue for relatively small numbers of patients in the United States, but they have been more common in the United Kingdom, where 1,300 severely ill psychiatric patients were brought to surgery from the late 1970s to the 1990s. Most of these patients had severe depression that was unresponsive to the standard fare, and a significant number had OCD.

Scientists such as Suzanne Haber of the University of Rochester Medical Center and Emory's Mahlon DeLong had been figuring out the organization of the basal ganglia and knew that this circuitry links to limbic regions that control emotion and behavior. Many Parkinson's patients also experience cognitive problems, including depression. Haber found that the cortico-basal ganglia-thalamic system involves a number of basic human behaviors, including reward, motivation, cognition, and motor control, and this involvement could be the key to linking Parkinson's and depression.

Major depression is very common; it affects about 8 percent of people in the United States and throughout the world each year. Patients can experience a range of symptoms, including apathy, an inability to feel pleasure, unshakable low moods, appetite and weight disturbances, exhaustion, impaired concentration, and suicidal ideation and behavior. Many people with major depression have multiple episodes, and it can affect all aspects of their lives. The World Health Organization's Global Burden of Disease Study, initiated in 1990, found that depression was the fourth leading cause of disability in the world, and the leading cause of disability in adults.[26]

Despite the fact that more than twenty drugs are approved for the treatment of depression, it can often take many medication trials to alleviate symptoms. And even among patients who have tried more than two drugs, 20 percent do not find relief. Some patients even undergo electroshock therapy without much effect. In 2005, 32,000 people in the United States killed themselves, and many times that number made an attempt. In many suicide cases, untreated depression is a major cause. Scientists have been working hard to understand the biology of the disease in an attempt to develop more targeted, effective treatments.

One of the first striking associations between depression and Parkinson's emerged quite by accident. In 2001, a French physician and scientist, Yves Agid, reported in the *New England Journal of Medicine* that electrical stimulation of the subthalamic nucleus accidentally turned on nearby nerve fibers that connect to the limbic system, the network of brain areas that control mood.[27] In one patient with Parkinson's disease, deep brain stimulation triggered an overwhelming feeling of sadness and despair. It went away when the stimulator was turned off. A CAT scan showed that the electrode was located close to the subthalamic nucleus, actually in the substantia nigra.

By the time Agid's report appeared in the prestigious journal, a neurologist named Helen Mayberg had spent almost fifteen years studying the brain circuits that underlie depression. Mayberg had pioneered functional mapping of the depressed brain at the University of Texas Health Sciences Center in San Antonio and before that at Johns Hopkins University School of Medicine. "I am using this disease to find the normal systems in the brain," she said. First, she mapped the depressed brain on medications, then on therapy, and then on a placebo pill. Each step of the way, she carefully mapped the brain as if it were a city of streets and avenues.

Mayberg thought depression offered the best hope of understanding the inner workings of the human brain, and so her focus had always been on the range of symptoms, stages, and treatments of severely depressed patients. She made it her business to know what the brain was up to when it was ill—when it was making the body slow down, cry, stay in bed, starve, sleep, and want to die. She realized that treatments took different roads within the brain, but they ultimately arrived at the same address. That's why people with depression could get better many different ways, even with a placebo pill.

The so-called limbic structures that regulate mood feed into the frontal cortex, the striatum, the thalamus, the hypothalamus, and the brain stem. These regions talk to one another all the time; thus, problems in the circuit could lead to difficulty with thinking, attention, mood, and behavior. Mayberg found that these circuits—particularly a hyperactive network of brain cells in the subgenual cingulate region, also called Brodmann area 25—are abnormally overactive in people with depression. Brodmann area 25 is "a big blob under the corpus callosum," explains Mayberg, who has mapped this region on thousands of brain scans. "This region talks to the cortex, the hypothalamus, and other regions involved in mood and behavior. The tracts travel in and out of this region," she says. "You can piece together the anatomy—the roadways—and see that they are all connecting to the subgenual cingulate."

When treatments work, the activity of these networks appears to return to normal. It makes sense that so many brain areas are involved in depression, which is not just negative mood. People lose their motivation to get out of bed, to work, to love. They have problems paying attention and thinking clearly. Their eating and sleeping patterns are way off-kilter.

For Mayberg, deep brain stimulation was the next logical step in figuring out how the network was broken in depression patients. In the late 1990s, she approached neurosurgeon Andres Lozano of the

University of Toronto, who was well known for his work in movement disorders. Mayberg wondered if deep brain stimulation could alter mood and behavior as well.

Lozano would be an ideal collaborator. He had arrived at the University of Toronto in 1991, a neurosurgeon with a postdoctoral degree in experimental medicine, and he had learned about deep brain stimulation from his mentor, Dr. Ronald Tasker, one of Canada's preeminent neurosurgeons. Tasker had helped usher in the field of functional stereotactic neurosurgery, and Lozano also learned how to do ablative surgery from him. They had already performed plenty of ablative operations and had implanted electrodes in the brains of patients with unrelenting pain, which was Tasker's real interest.

But Tasker was also well known for his fine maps of the human thalamus and brain stem, and he had performed a few DBS implants for patients with movement disorders in the late 1980s, after Benabid. In 1992, Lozano and his colleagues used deep brain stimulation on their first Parkinson's patient. Five years later, they used the technique for dystonia. The Canadian group then led the way from dystonia to epilepsy, and ultimately into the work Mayberg would invite them to do on depression.

"These are the circuits for depression," Mayberg told Lozano, as she pulled out a scan of the depressed brain. "Can we do something about it?" Lozano was intrigued and said that he thought it was well worth trying.

"I didn't see any difference between psychiatric symptoms or neurological ones," said Lozano. He believes that neurosurgeons today have followed a path that Wilder Penfield laid out for them fifty years ago. "It is Penfield revisited," he said of this expanding exploration of the brain's electrical circuits. But this time, investigators had modern scientific tools to guide them and to study what they were doing.

Thus, in 1999, Mayberg moved to the University of Toronto ready to devise and test deep brain stimulation in severely depressed patients for whom nothing else was working. In 2002, the team was granted approval to operate on six patients. They brought their first one into the operating room a year later, in 2003. They worked with a whole team of specialists—psychiatrists, psychologists, neurologists, and ethicists—to figure out who should be allowed entry into the study.

"This became a proof-of-principle experiment," Mayberg said. Using deep brain stimulation to treat intractable depression would help prove her finding about the abnormal activity of the networks that she had documented on the brain scans. What's more, the team would follow the DBS patients over time to figure out whether the treatment worked for those with such severe depression—and, if so, *how* it worked.

When Mayberg, Lozano, and their colleagues were ready for their first patient in 2003, their target for the electrodes was Brodmann area 25, which Mayberg had found in her earlier studies to be abnormally overactive in depressed patients.

Deanna Cole-Benjamin, a public health nurse, was the sixth patient at the University of Toronto to undergo deep brain stimulation for severe and unrelenting depression. Virtually every antidepressant on the market, as well as eighty rounds of electroshock therapy, had failed her. "It was worse than being dead in a way," said Cole-Benjamin. Her suicidal thoughts and actions had led to four years in and out of the Kingston Psychiatric Hospital, a massive collection of stone buildings with bars on the windows and locks on the doors on Lake Ontario in Canada.

"I will not leave a stone unturned," promised Dr. Gebrehiwot Abraham, a soft-spoken psychiatrist who had followed her care at the hospital. He kept his word. He heard about an experimental surgery to implant electrodes into the brain to stimulate abnormal networks in patients with severe depression, and Cole-Benjamin proved to be a perfect candidate.

Mayberg was at Cole-Benjamin's side as Lozano operated on her. Cole-Benjamin was so profoundly ill that she could barely talk. Lozano turned up the device to stimulate the first contact. Nothing. When Lozano turned up the stimulation more, the patient described a brighter feeling. When he turned it off, she fell quiet again and thought maybe it was just her imagination.

"In truth, we didn't know what to expect," said Mayberg. "We just didn't want something bad to happen. This was a test of an idea that needed to be done ethically, safely, and in the right people. If it had been at all ambiguous, I would have said stop. But this was not subtle at all. This was one of those *aha!* moments that we could not have imagined. We had no expectations that depression could have any acute elements. We thought that the scans over time would tell the story if the device worked."

To Mayberg, the most salient observation was that the patients seemed to gain access to their former selves again. She thought that might be the key to understanding what these brain circuits actually do. "These patients have been ill for a very long time. It's become adaptive, but not functionally adaptive. You have to retrain them the same way you would if you are healing from a bad hip. You replace the hip but you don't go out the next day and run a marathon."

Within a few weeks, the symptoms that had plagued Cole-Benjamin for four years were significantly decreased. Before her surgery, she told Mayberg that she wanted to be able to hug her children and to feel their warmth and love. Finally, after years of hiding under her covers, she could hug her children and feel deep pleasure.

Others in the study got better over time as well. Lozano and Mayberg's patent is now in the hands of Advanced Neuromodulation Systems, a company that tests implantable therapies for chronic pain and neurological disorders and is part of the technology firm St. Jude Medical. In April 2008, the company announced a multicenter study to test DBS for depression.

Around the same time, Benjamin Greenberg and his team at Brown University were also thinking about depression. They had had success with deep brain stimulation for obsessive-compulsive disorder, and many of their patients had reported changes in mood. This had the team wondering about the possibility of tackling depression with the electrodes. The Brown/Clevelend collaboration had by then expanded to include scientists at Harvard's Massachusetts General Hospital. They got together to talk about how they would go about designing and carrying out a study on some of the country's most depressed patients.

Greenberg's experience with DBS in OCD patients was based on stimulating a different area of the brain from Mayberg and Lozano's Brodmann area 25. Instead, the Brown/Cleveland/Harvard team was a veteran squad working in and around the basal ganglia. For OCD, they had implanted electrodes into the ventral internal capsule/ventral striatum, a region that is located in front of the anterior commissure and includes parts of the nucleus accumbens and the red nucleus. This was where they wanted to go with bilateral electrode implants for depression. The area is rich in serotonin, long associated with depression, and it contains white matter fibers that link the orbitofrontal cortex, the mesiofrontal cortex, and the dorsolateral frontal cortex to the thalamus, the hypothalamus, the amygdala, and the brain stem—all structures involved in depression. And, as Lozano would explain, both of these targets—area 25 and the VC/VS—could work because they are like interconnected highways that use different routes to reach the same destinations.

In 2002, all three hospitals had the IRB approvals in place to test the stimulators for the treatment of depression, and in January 2003 Greenberg and his colleagues at Brown brought their first patient into the operating room. The Cleveland Clinic team followed shortly thereafter, and then in 2004 the Harvard group began implanting DBS for depression.

One of the Harvard group's patients was thirty-three-year-old Melissa Murphy. When she arrived at psychiatrist Darin Dougherty's office at Mass General, Dougherty was almost two years into the depression study but was still looking for patients who could pass the strict entry qualifications. Candidates had to have tried and failed at least ten trials of medications, as well as bilateral electroshock therapy, and Murphy had done all that.

Depression had landed in Murphy's life with no warning two years earlier, when the happily married and successful public relations executive got up from her desk on a warm summer afternoon, walked out of her office, and never returned. She went home and cried, and she had no idea why. Other than for an occasional doctor's appointment, she did not shower or dress for the outside world for months. Her husband, Scott, had taken a job in Boston and she had remained in Chicago. For a while, she kept up appearances on the phone with Scott. Deeply, painfully depressed, she remained in this numb state until October, when Scott traveled to Chicago, packed her up, and moved her back east.

By then, Murphy's weight had dropped below one hundred pounds. Neither the therapists she saw four times a week nor all the medicine she took for months on end helped her. Realizing how bad things really were, her family arranged for her to undergo electroshock therapy, but despite seventeen sessions—to both sides of the brain—"Nothing made a dent," Murphy recalled.

Finally, she became suicidal. One day she swallowed an entire month's supply of the antianxiety drug Klonopin. Scott Murphy picked up his blond-haired, blue-eyed high school sweetheart, carried her to the car, and headed for the emergency room of a local hospital. After five days at a small psychiatric residence, there was talk of hospitalizing her in a locked unit at nearby McLean Hospital, but Melissa Murphy was petrified when she saw a patient restrained in her bed. She begged her husband to take her home.

Melissa and Scott had been married for six years. After she became depressed, he never felt she was safe unless he was home, watching her. The medical bills were piling up to the tune of thousands of dollars a week. The house was a wreck. "Promise me you'll be safe," was Scott Murphy's daily mantra to his wife.

Murphy would burn herself with cigarettes to see what it felt like. Another time her husband found her eyeing the blade of a circular saw in the basement. She took kitchen knives to cut her wrists. She was hospitalized, released, and admitted a second time. Her husband escorted her to a locked ward, but she cried and cried, and he finally argued with the staff to let him take her home.

By the time Murphy showed up at Dougherty's office, she had been treated by six other psychiatrists. He looked at a summary of all the treatments and thought about trying vagus nerve stimulation, which recently had been approved for treatment-resistant depression. The vagus nerve starts at the brain stem and descends to the neck, chest, and abdomen. It helps in sensing aortic blood pressure, slowing heart rate, stimulating digestive organs, and managing taste. Studies show that the nerve projects to some areas of the brain associated with depression, and for still unexplained reasons, stimulating it seems to lift mood in about a third of patients. Surgeons thread a wire into the neck, wrap it around the nerve, and connect the wire to a battery-operated pacemaker in the chest. But

Dougherty felt that Murphy was too sick for even vagus nerve stimulation to help.

"I had never seen anything like it," said Dougherty. "She was completely shut down. She spoke very softly and slowly and she was very confused." Murphy needed something more powerful.

Murphy became the tenth patient to undergo deep brain stimulation in the Cleveland, Brown, and Harvard collaboration. Dougherty set a date in July 2006, but the team moved the surgery up because they realized that it was indeed a life-and-death matter.

On the eve of the operation, Murphy had a splitting headache. Only her husband would know about it; she didn't want to give up her spot in the operating room. Dougherty stood at her side in the operating room; Emad Eskandar was the neurosurgeon. Greenberg had come in from Rhode Island as well. As they looked at the scans of Murphy's brain pinned to the light box on the wall, they focused on her ventral capsule/ventral striatum, their target, with its large fiber bundles connecting the thalamus to the orbital and medial prefrontal cortex.

During the operation, the team waited for some sign that the leads were in the right place. They sent high-frequency stimulation to the electrode and looked for a response indicating a lift in Murphy's mood. Mayberg and Lozano had reported these acute signs of change, and Rezai and his team had seen it as well. Some depressed patients smiled on the operating table for the first time in decades; some reported a deep connectedness they hadn't felt in years. Then the device would be shut off, and their worlds would go dark again, at least until the second phase of the procedure to implant the batteries in the chest wall, connect the leads, and begin the long and challenging task of programming. But Murphy doesn't remember any clouds parting in the operating room.

The next day, Murphy was under general anesthesia when they placed two small batteries on either side of her chest. Three weeks later, she returned to Dougherty's office, where Greenberg turned on the batteries and began programming the device. And Melissa Murphy laughed for the first time in years.

During Murphy's programming with Greenberg, she remembers feeling a rush of warm blood throughout her body right before she laughed. When the stimulator was turned off, the warmth was gone. She was nervous. She wasn't sure how she was supposed to act. She didn't want to screw things up. Was she going to fail? Were they going to be disappointed? What she remembers most about that day was that her body felt literally lighter, though she was then a mere ninety-eight pounds.

Programming is part art, part science. It is also time-consuming; it generally can take a few hours a day over several days, but many patients have returned dozens of times over many months, even years, for readjustments. Psychiatrist Donald Malone of Cleveland Clinic, who does the macrostimulation and programming for deep brain stimulation, tests each of the four contacts by turning on the stimulating electrode and painstakingly asking the patient to report what he or she is experiencing moment by moment. Some contacts can bring on anxiety, warmth, sweating, or even sadness. "I test each one to titrate and evaluate the setting. I find the one that is right, the one that gives the patient the right mix of better mood without overdoing it. This is very labor-intensive," Malone explained.

Murphy's initial setting was four volts on each side, and it was later increased to eight volts. The team constantly used depression rating scores to evaluate the effects of the treatment. The change was slow and steady, and the battery seemed to need changing every six months—each change meaning another day of surgery to open up Murphy's chest and slip in a new battery. (Companies that manufacturer these devices say that the batteries should last up to five years.) And she has had to go back many times for reprogramming of the stimulators. "Oh, but it's worth it," Murphy said, a year into the treatment. "I love my settings now. It just makes it easier to be me again. I have an outlook. I have goals."

Murphy wanted to focus more on her husband, to reach out to friends and family, to find a job, to experience gratitude, and to start running again. But how far could she come back? Deep brain stimulation turned out to be something less than the instant cure that Murphy—like most people who were undergoing the treatment—hoped it would be. "I thought that once they turned it on I would be better right away," Murphy said. "But it has taken a lot longer than I thought." She still had great difficulty with concentration, memory, and thinking clearly. Doctors kept records of these symptoms because it was possible that they were side effects of the device itself.

Patients like Murphy truly put deep brain stimulation to the test. Almost eighteen months after the stimulators were turned on, she was still not working. "December was just so bleak and dreary and seemingly endless," she wrote in her journal at the start of 2007. "All the questions around life still linger." She felt that the holiday season was hard, and she was lonely. "I am trying so hard," she said. A week later, she noted the joy she felt with her dog, Ned, asleep at her feet and her husband in the same state of slumber by her side. "I must partake in this joy because that is what it is: joy."

It is still not clear whether deep brain stimulation works for patients like Murphy. Many are doing better after a year, but it is still too early in the studies to draw a conclusion. It certainly doesn't work for everybody. But Greenberg said he hopes DBS can ultimately help some of the patients whom psychiatrists have been unable to treat conventionally. "Stimulating this network affects motivation, social interaction, the ability to experience pleasure and anxiety," Greenberg explained. "You often hear people saying that the room looks brighter, that a weight has lifted" when the stimulators are tested during the surgery.

But Greenberg has learned to temper his expectations; as he discovered, the human brain has a long history of recording memory and mood, and it will take more than just one click of a button and a turn of a dial to get people better. While it is exciting to see patients smile or laugh in the operating room, "We have learned not to go overboard," said Greenberg. "These are people who haven't lived with normal affect for a very long time. They may not have a recent experience of it. You don't want to give them a sense that smiling and laughing is a constant mood state. But you want to be able to restore their capacity for smiling and laughing."

By January 2008, twenty-eight patients with severe depression had had deep brain stimulation surgery in Toronto, and nine had undergone the procedure at Emory University, where Mayberg had moved to continue her work in DBS for depression. Seventeen had been through the Brown/ Cleveland/Harvard study.[28] While Mayberg and Lozano were working with Advanced Neuromodulation Systems, Medtronic was planning a multicenter trial to study DBS for depression in collaboration with the Brown/Cleveland/Harvard group and others.

The preliminary work in the Brown collaboration showed that their first sixteen patients had improved by about 50 percent at the one-year follow-up. And this was after a lot of readjusting of the stimulators to find the right balance to help alleviate the symptoms. Analysis of the Toronto/ Emory results also found that deep brain stimulation was successful in about 60 percent of severely depressed patients.[29] And even when it didn't totally do the job, patients wanted to keep the stimulators in place.

Mayberg has made it her life's work to understand how deep brain stimulation circumvents depression. She wants to know what stimulation at 130 hertz does to the brain network involved, and what clues it might give to why people get depression in the first place. She also wants to know whether the procedure affects sleep and, if so, how. She wants to understand the behavioral phenomena—the acute smiling or laughing or feeling of connectedness—that occur in the operating room. As this book is being written, Mayberg is testing whether two electrodes, one on each side of the brain, are necessary. Perhaps one would do the trick. And maybe it isn't necessary to go to 130 hertz to return these patients to a more normal mood. Maybe 60 hertz would work.

It is still not clear what deep brain stimulation is actually doing at the network level. Mayberg believes that this depression network is overactive, but teams of scientists have shown that stimulation activates output from the brain network involved in depression. According to Jerry Vitek, now at the Cleveland Clinic, stimulation not only activates the output from the stimulated structure but also changes the pattern of neuronal activity from a noisy, chaotic signal to a more regular one. Vitek believes that this may be the key to how it works, but notes that much remains to be done to understand the effects on the network and how it may change with long-term stimulation.

Mayberg is taking the steps to study and address these issues. "This is highly selective modulation," she said. "It gives us important clues where to shine the light."

In 2008, deep brain stimulation for depression was still very much an experimental procedure, and the mechanisms underlying the clinical changes in patients remained a mystery. "We want to treat depression like we treat heart disease," said Mayberg, who received research funds from private foundations, including the Dana Foundation, the Stanley Foundation, and the Woodruff Foundation (through Emory University). Her initial discoveries on the networks involved in depression were funded by the National Alliance for Research in Depression and Schizophrenia.

Additional studies and meticulous analysis of the results are necessary. "It doesn't help patients to be led on unless there is good data," Mayberg said.

Chapter 8

Tourette Syndrome

I f any brain condition captures the complexity of the abnormal brain under fire from both ends of the spectrum—from movement to behavior—it is Tourette syndrome.

The disorder takes its name from Georges Albert Édouard Brutus Gilles de la Tourette, born in 1857 in Saint Gervais-les-Trois-Clochers, France. After completing his medical studies, the young doctor began working with one of the most influential neurologists of his day, Jean-Martin Charcot. Tourette was interested in psychotherapy, hypnosis, and hysteria. These interests led him to see a handful of young people with what was first called "la maladie des tics," the common symptoms of which were both motor and verbal problems, such as repetitive eye blinking or shrugs and meaningless sounds or blurted-out words or phrases. Tourette began using hypnosis in an effort to cure these patients, but it didn't work.

The physician had his own series of maladies. He lost his son and was said to have developed mood swings that ended his career and forced him to live his last two years in a psychiatric hospital in Switzerland. Tourette was forty-seven when he died.

At the turn of the twentieth century, Sigmund Freud said that Tourette syndrome patients suffered neurosis, and the screaming, barking, and foul language represented underlying hostile feelings. Talk therapy did not work, however. Others believed that the symptoms were signs of being possessed by the devil. It is thought that people with both Tourette syndrome and Huntington's disease were probably subjected to exorcism rites in witch-burning days.

In 1965, things began to change slowly. A young psychiatrist named Arthur Shapiro in New York was asked to see a patient with tics—her head, shoulders, eyes, and tongue were constantly in motion. She was a well-dressed, quiet, working girl, but without warning she would uncontrollably utter vulgar four-letter words. Mortified and ashamed, she looked to this young doctor for help.

The case puzzled Shapiro. His patient seemed quite normal. She just wanted to get rid of her symptoms. He found a name for her condition in a medical book—Gilles de la Tourette's disease—but there were no effective treatments listed. In the 1960s, Shapiro diagnosed a thirteen-year-old patient with Tourette syndrome and began experimenting with a host of new drugs available for psychiatric patients. He happened on haloperidol, a drug that was used to reduce the symptoms of psychosis. It was the same drug that Rob Weil, the physician ultimately diagnosed with dystonia, was given when a doctor mistakenly thought he had Tourette.

The drug alleviated virtually all the tics in Shapiro's patient. "I really felt like a doctor for the first time. I cured someone," Shapiro said decades later. "Psychological treatments took so long and the effects were so subtle. Here was a drug that immediately got rid of these horrible symptoms."

At the time, only fifty or so cases had been reported in the medical literature worldwide. Word spread that Shapiro, along with his wife, Elaine, worked with Tourette patients. Today, Tourette syndrome experts say that as many as 250,000 people in the United States have the classic symptoms of the disorder. If transient or chronic motor tics are included, the incidence is much higher. In recent years, researchers have found evidence that the humming, swearing, barking, and sniffling may be caused by an excess of the brain chemical dopamine, which also has been implicated in schizophrenia and other psychiatric disorders. (People with Parkinson's disease have the opposite problem: they have depleted stores of dopamine cells in the regions that involve movement.) Drugs that block dopamine stop both motor and vocal tics in people with Tourette, but the medicines do not work for all patients.

Scientists have long believed that Tourette syndrome is predominantly a genetically based disorder, since it runs in families. The vocal and motor tics are more prominent in males, as is the condition itself. On the other hand, females in Tourette families are more likely to have symptoms of obsessive-compulsive disorder. Many Tourette patients also suffer from attention-deficit/hyperactivity disorder. The symptoms of Tourette generally appear in childhood. For unknown reasons, the symptoms appear to burn out by adulthood in many patients, although some spend a lifetime disabled by the condition. A long list of medications has been tried on patients, as well as behavioral treatments. Some patients who have found no relief have ended up in the operating room.

Neurosurgeons started operating on the worst cases of Tourette syndrome in the mid-1950s, and in the ensuing years the procedures and their targets have been diverse, including prefrontal lobotomy. But surgeons have also gone after limbic structures via surgical techniques called limbic leucotomy and anterior cingulotomy. Lesions to the thalamus and the cerebellum have also been tried. In 2003, Yasin Temel and Veerle Visser-Vandewalle of the Academic Hospital Maastricht, Netherlands, reported on a sweep they conducted of the literature from 1960 to 2003. Their review of twenty-four reports covering sixty-five patients found that the results had often been unsatisfactory or had resulted in partial paralysis or even dystonia.

The first deep brain stimulation surgery for Tourette syndrome took place in 1999. By 2003, when Vandewalle reported the results of the literature review at a Movement Disorders Society meeting, only three Tourette patients had been fitted with stimulating electrodes. The reports on those patients, who had undergone bilateral thalamic stimulation, were that the treatment was showing "promising results on tics and obsessive-compulsive symptoms."[30]

But scientists also had reason to believe that stimulation elsewhere in the neighborhood of the thalamus could be helpful. After all,

Tourette was a type of movement disorder, even if its physical process was unknown, and structures in and around the basal ganglia had long served as targets, often with good results, for movement disorders. In 2005, scientists at Massachusetts General Hospital selected a white matter area (called the anterior limb of the internal capsule) near the thalamus and a portion of the basal ganglia for the treatment of a forty-year-old woman who had suffered from disabling vocalizations and severe head and arm jerking since she was ten. Her symptoms were so severe that they resulted in blindness in one eye. She had been given more than forty medicines and other therapies to relieve the tics, but nothing had worked. On the basis of studies they were doing on obsessive-compulsive disorder and depression, the investigators hoped that deep brain stimulation would help her.

Neurosurgeon Emad Eskandar and his colleagues implanted bilateral electrodes in the anterior limb of the internal capsule, ending in the vicinity of the nucleus accumbens. After they found the right levels for the frequency and voltage, the patient's symptoms were substantially reduced. Eighteen months later, she was still doing better than she had been, but then her surgeons found that the electrodes had been damaged. They removed the electrodes and replaced them with thalamic stimulators. The change resulted in significantly better control of her tics.[31]

In the nineteenth century, Tourette and Charcot were sure that the syndrome was organic, but they had to deduce from psychological experiments such as hypnosis that it was not purely mental. Modern researchers were better off in that they could use new imaging technology to look into the brain, and with talk of electrode stimulation as a potentially effective treatment, the challenge was to figure out just where the DBS electrodes should go. A team of scientists from Weill Cornell Medical Center in New York City brought six men with the syndrome into their laboratory for brain scan studies to identify the functional neuroanatomy of the condition. David Silbersweig and his wife, Emily Stern, both physicians, and their colleagues used a machine called a positron-emission tomography scanner and found more than a dozen abnormally active brain regions. They concluded that the aberrant activity in the sensorimotor, language, executive, and paralimbic circuits accounted for the "initiation and execution of diverse motor and vocal behaviors." The study was published in the *Archives of General Psychiatry* in 2000.[32]

A group of Italian researchers has done much of the work on deep brain stimulation for Tourette. Domenico Servello is a neurosurgeon at the Hospital of Galeazzi in Milan, Italy. After studying the various brain regions targeted during surgery for Tourette, Sevello and his team touched down on the centromedian thalamus. In 1999, they began identifying patients who had not responded to at least six months of standard treatments. The team amassed a large series of eighteen patients who underwent bilateral deep brain surgery with the leads placed on both sides of the thalamus, in the centromedian-parafascicular and ventralis oralis complex. They then assessed the patients at least every three months for up to eighteen months. To varying degrees, all responded to the stimulation. Many of their disabling symptoms—obsessive-compulsive disorder, self-injurious behaviors, anxiety, and tics—decreased after the electrodes were turned on and adjusted. The results of the study were published in the *Journal of Neurology and Neurosurgery* in 2008.

All this work was exciting, but, as is usually the case in experimental medicine, the possible use of deep brain stimulation for Tourette was kept generally confined to the research world. That changed in 2004 when Robert Maciunas, a neurosurgeon at University Hospitals in Cleveland, brought a young man named Jeffrey Matovic into surgery to implant electrodes. A few weeks later, on April 1, clips of the operation were shown to the nation over morning coffee on ABC's *Good Morning America*. Matovic was the first American patient with Tourette to be treated with deep brain stimulation.[33]

The national Tourette Syndrome Association (TSA) worked quickly to control the buzz in the Tourette community. Neurologist Jonathan W. Mink of the University of Rochester Medical Center, a scientific advisor to the association, found himself trying to dissuade patients and family members from seeking out the expensive and experimental surgical technique. Little was known about the benefits of the surgery, and more important, no one knew who would even be a candidate. Ethics was a major issue, as many patients develop the condition in early childhood and symptoms lessen significantly with age. Mink was worried that desperate parents would bring their children into surgery without waiting to see if time itself would alleviate the symptoms.

It wasn't clear that deep brain stimulation worked, and if it did, no one knew exactly why. Mink pointed to the risks associated with the surgical treatment, including brain bleeds, infection, and stroke. And all sorts of side effects had been reported from experiments with the technique in other brain conditions, including changes in mood, motor function, sensation, and cognition.

The TSA issued a statement from Mink and other TSA scientific advisors: "It should be noted that this is a single case report involving one patient with TS. ... While it is encouraging that at the present time the patient is experiencing a reduction in symptoms, insufficient time has elapsed since the operation to conclude that this symptom abatement will persist."

By 2005, the TSA advisors had developed a set of recommendations. A year later, they held a workshop on DBS in Stresa, Italy, to learn what they could from the Milan team that had the most experience with deep brain stimulation for the condition. The recommendations were published in *Movement Disorders* in November 2006. They generated a list of symptoms that should disqualify patients from DBS, including tics due to other causes; other medical, neurological, or psychiatric disorders that might preclude full participation in DBS treatment; the likelihood that patients would need and benefit from psychological intervention; psychosocial factors that would preclude full participation in DBS; and determination of a person's willingness to participate in psychological interventions for psychosocial problems. The group also concluded that teams should wait until a Tourette patient has reached adulthood in order to avoid operating on people whose symptoms might get better by the time they reach their twenties.

But Irving Cooper—Coop the King—would have been proud. The publicity genie was already out of the bottle: on March 13, 2006, not one but two nationally televised programs about deep brain stimulation for

Tourette aired, beating the TSA's November recommendations by eight months. The shows themselves were a tale of two ways to publish research in the popular media. One was blasted by alarmed Tourette experts who said that the technique's benefit was oversimplified. The report omitted or minimized the unknowns about Tourette and the risks of deep brain stimulation. The other, which received warm praise for accuracy and sobriety, was a segment on the Discovery Health Channel's *Medical Incredible* series. This was the story of Steve Blackman, a fifty-year-old EMS technician who had suffered from severe Tourette most of his life and who had become the second person in the United States to have DBS surgery for the syndrome.

Steve Blackman's phone buzzed after the *Good Morning America* segment on Jeffrey Martovic's surgery. Blackman's symptoms, which had started when he was a toddler, included twitching, eye blinking, grunting, and "the whole shebang of symptoms" characteristic of Tourette. Although for decades he had been able to work as an emergency medical technician and was able to suppress his tics when he took care of patients, things had grown worse, and eventually he had to give up his job. The dozen medicines he had to take to control all of his symptoms—as well as the pain triggered by decades of violent movements of his neck and spine—left him unable to drive a car, let alone an ambulance. A former nurse called to tell him about the Matovic piece, and Blackman immediately called his psychiatrist, James Leckman at the Yale Child Study Center, who is considered one of the world's leading experts on Tourette.

"Steve," Leckman said, "if you're not a candidate, no one is." Blackman was one of Leckman's most challenging patients.

While Blackman's symptoms began at the age of three, it had taken ten years for a diagnosis, during which time embarrassing vocal tics, screaming, grunting, and all sorts of noises had emerged from his mouth. It was 1969, and teachers made him stand in the corner, with the tics growing worse as his classmates stared. At home, his father beat him and made him write thousands of times over, "I will not tic." By his sophomore year in high school, his mother had taken him to the Mayo Clinic. She had tried everything. At the Mayo Clinic, he was put on a ward with teenagers who had all sorts of psychiatric problems. They fed him heavy doses of the antipsychotic drug Haldol. The ward was complete with its own padded room, which Blackman saw only from the outside.

As he got older, Blackman's tics were so violent that his head jerked in different directions. It led to spinal stenosis and injuries to his body. "The pain was incredible. My bones and my muscles were damaged," he said years later. One side of his body was shorter than the other, and he wore a brace on his leg. He was prone to falling because of the way his body had grown into the tics. His two dogs bolstered him when he slipped and remained his constant companions.

Blackman would count the number of tics he had in one day. On many days, he hit two thousand, even in adulthood.

In July 2004, Yale neurosurgeon Alain de Lotbinière performed DBS surgery on Blackman. The surgeon and Leckman were nervous, and rightly so. There was virtually no scientific evidence for efficacy of DBS for Tourette syndrome, and going inside Blackman's brain was a little like exploratory surgery in the bigger sense of the word. They hoped that things would be better, but they had no idea whether brain stimulation to the thalamus would do the job.

Blackman's body was so out of control that he had to be put under general anesthesia for the entire procedure. (It is usually done while patients are sedated but awake enough to respond to questions.) They didn't turn the stimulator on for three weeks, but the surgery itself had a positive effect on Blackman's symptoms: he didn't have one tic during that entire stretch of time. Not one.

As do a small minority of patients with Tourette syndrome, Blackman suffered from coprolalia, the involuntary blurting out of curse words. He also would hear a phrase in his brain and keep repeating it out loud. This is called echolalia. These symptoms disappeared in the months following the activation of the stimulator. But the tics returned. Blackman continued to count them, and they decreased in number every day. The tics were down to ninety-five on a good day. On a not-so-good day they might reach a count of two hundred.

DBS wasn't working as well as Blackman had hoped. He got some help from Joan Miravite, a nurse practitioner who worked with DBS patients. She called herself a professional hand-holder. The job suited her; in time, Medtronic hired her as an associate therapy consultant to teach doctors how to program the device and to call on patients such as Blackman. She would do regular checkups on their symptoms and the settings of the stimulators. When things weren't going well, she would program Blackman's device herself.

As DBS innovators had found with Parkinson's, dystonia, and OCD, getting the programming just right for each patient was the key. The goal was to obtain all the possible benefits while minimizing side effects. And each manifestation of the disorder brought its unique problems. Blackman was still very disabled, still unable to work. He wanted more benefit than the device could offer, and he traveled to his surgeon's office many times for readjustment of the device. Sometimes it made things worse; other times he would get better for a while and then slide back into his symptoms. Some other DBS patients he met had had their devices removed, but he wasn't giving up.

About three years into the treatment, Blackman and his doctors talked about the possibility of more surgery to add an additional set of electrodes in another brain region, perhaps the globus pallidus. But identifying the right target was difficult. The parameters for the surgery came from studying Tourette patients who had undergone DBS, and by that time there were still only about twenty-five in the United States and fewer than a hundred worldwide. Today, Blackman averages around a hundred tics a day, but all the symptoms of screaming, cursing, and repeating of words are gone.

"The best move of my life was having this surgery," he said. "I knew how dangerous it was. I knew the risks. But I couldn't go on the way I was."

The other show that aired on March 13, 2006, was a segment on another ABC network program, *Miracle Workers*, a medical reality show. This one was all Hollywood. It illustrated the kind of careless hype that the TSA feared and sought to ward off. It told of deep brain surgery performed on a teenager with Tourette syndrome at Tulane University in New Orleans.

In early 2005, Dr. Donald Richardson, a seventy-four-year-old neuro-surgeon at Tulane, operated on nineteen-year-old Emily Bresler. Richardson had been part of an old and controversial history. The founder of Tulane's psychiatric department, Robert Heath, was a leader in the first generation of neurosurgeons who destroyed tissue in the brains of psychiatric patients—most infamously, African Americans—to alter their behavior and mood.

Emily Bresler had spent most of her life making involuntary move-ments and blurting out curse words. Sometimes her hands had a violent life of their own, and she would smack herself in the head. Richardson had been using modern-day deep brain stimulation tools since the 1970s. He had implanted electrodes for chronic pain, Parkinson's, essential tremor, and dystonia and had already given implants to his first Tourette syndrome patient, a thirty-one-year-old man from Mississippi.

When he operated on Bresler, Richardson performed the surgery in two phases, just as neurosurgeons were doing for other deep brain stimu-lation surgeries. He implanted electrodes in each side of the brain, and the thalamus was his target. A day later, he implanted two battery-operated stimulator devices in Bresler's chest. The surgeries were filmed so they could be aired on *Miracle Workers*.

To a reporter from the *Tulane University Magazine*, Richardson explained his embracing of the new DBS technique in the context of his personal history: "I did procedures on Tourette patients years ago, before we had a stimulator. ... What we found is that if we put an electrode in the brain, found the right spot and stimulated it, we could markedly make the patient's Tourette symptoms worse. Then, if we made a small lesion and coagulated that area, the symptoms got much better." But his tech-nique didn't hold up, he said, and he stopped doing it. Then modern deep brain stimulation came along, and Richardson opened the gate again: "I think the future for deep-brain stimulation is almost limitless. We're just scratching the surface."[34]

As of 2007, the number of cases of DBS for Tourette in the medical liter-ature was growing, and the brain targets varied. There was an increasing number of teenagers in the operating room as well, despite the TSA advi-sory group's recommendations.[35]

Chapter 9

Battling Epilepsy

A s surgeons and neurologists used deep brain stimulation to tackle a wide array of vexing brain problems, it came as no surprise that epilepsy soon found itself on the DBS radar. After all, it was Wilder Penfield who first used stimulating electrodes in his epilepsy patients to help identify the locations of the seizures. Now, almost fifty years later, scientists were debating just how to bring DBS to patients with intractable epilepsy. One idea was to do deep brain stimulation to keep electrical activity of the brain in check. The other idea was to suppress seizure activity by delivering electrical stimulation only when the brain "sensed" that a seizure was in the offing. Unlike the constant deep brain stimulation signal delivered for Parkinson's and other conditions, scientists would have to figure out a way to deliver this electrical signal only as needed, at the first neural hint of a seizure.

Epilepsy is relatively common, affecting 1 to 2 percent of the U.S. population. The range of seizures is very broad, from the almost imperceptible "absence" seizure, lasting only seconds, to the grand mal type, which can last as long as two minutes. Scientists have a fair idea of what the brain is doing in a seizure: brain cells communicate through electrical impulses, and when these signals misfire, the disturbance can cause chemical changes triggering a multitude of symptoms, such as confusion or temporary loss of consciousness. Many factors can lead to these electrical misfirings, including head trauma, brain tumors, strokes, and infections such as encephalitis. There are also genes that put people at risk for seizures. Despite all this information, however, doctors who treat epilepsy still have no way to explain why nearly 70 percent of their patients have seizures.

With more than a dozen epilepsy drugs on the market, doctors and their patients have worked hard to find the right mix to eliminate or reduce seizures with as few side effects as possible. Even so, only 50 to 75 percent of patients are seizure-free and unburdened by the sleepiness caused by the medicines. Surgery to remove the vulnerable tissue has been very successful at eliminating seizures, but that is useful only if the seizures arise from one particular area in the brain. Such seizures are called focal seizures, and only about half of epilepsy patients have them; the rest have generalized seizures, which are more widespread in the brain and more difficult to treat.

In the most commonly used surgical procedure for epilepsy, doctors remove tissue containing the cortical brain cells that give rise to the seizures. Surgeons can also use a gamma knife (a targeted beam of radiation) in lieu of a traditional surgical cut. In 1997, another approach came online when the FDA approved stimulators of the vagus nerve. These lessened, but usually did not eliminate, seizures in half the patients for whom nothing else worked.

Irving Cooper actually pioneered brain stimulation as a treatment for epilepsy in the early 1970s. He targeted the cerebellum, which is involved in controlling voluntary muscle movement, in thirty-two patients. Cooper reported improvements in less than half of the patients. He also became the first to try stimulation in the thalamus. He targeted a part of the thalamus called the anterior nucleus in six patients and reported that four improved.

In the late 1980s, a team of brothers at the National Medical Center and General Hospital in Mexico City—neurosurgeon Francisco Velasco and neurologist Marcos Velasco—moved to another spot in the thalamus, the centromedial nucleus. Between 1987 and 2001 they published a series of studies covering more than eighty patients. The studies seemed to make a good case for stimulating this region of the thalamus.[36]

Robert Fisher, director of the epilepsy center at Stanford University and one of the most distinguished neurologists in the country, knew about the Velascos' early work and decided to start his own experiments using stimulation to treat his epilepsy patients. The Velasco studies had been open-label—that is, both the researcher and the patient knew the treatment the patient was receiving. Fisher, whose study had only seven patients, made the test more rigorous; his not only was double-blind—with neither the researcher nor the participant knowing what treatment the patient was receiving—but also used a "crossover" design. This meant that at one point in the experiment all the subjects switched from the active treatment to a placebo or vice versa.

In 1992, Fisher and his colleagues reported their results. During the double-blind crossover period, the patients averaged about a 30 percent decrease in seizures when the stimulation was on.[37] It certainly wasn't an overwhelming success. But in the second part of the study, which was the open-label design, three of the patients did better. Their seizure frequency decreased by half. The researchers were perplexed, but they speculated that this result reflected a strong placebo effect.

Fisher headed back into the research laboratory to find a better target. In France, Benabid also had experience with epilepsy, with the subthalamic nucleus as his target, and said that he saw "dramatic improvement" in some patients and a much smaller benefit in others. Two other groups recently had reported similar experiences. With the results so mixed, it still wasn't clear how the device could best be used—there were questions about the exact tissue to stimulate as well as the frequency of the stimulation and how it should be delivered.

The most likely candidate was still the thalamus, the brain's major thoroughfare. All sensory information except smell goes through the thalamus before heading to the cortex. Fisher and others reasoned that stimulating the thalamus could influence the electrical activity over wide regions of cortex.

Reviewing the literature, they found themselves back where Cooper had left off almost decades earlier: in the anterior nucleus of the thalamus. By 2004, two groups in the United States—Fisher's in California and another in Pennsylvania—had tried deep brain stimulation of the anterior nucleus in their epilepsy patients. They found that it reduced the number of seizures by about 40 percent without any obvious side effects. Andres Lozano and his colleagues at the University of Toronto also had success stimulating the anterior thalamic nucleus in five epilepsy patients. A year after the DBS surgery, three of Lozano's five patients had 30 to 40 percent fewer seizures. One patient was virtually seizure-free.

Then, in 2006, Fisher began the largest study yet undertaken to assess the safety and effectiveness of deep brain stimulation for epilepsy, focusing on the region of the brain that was yielding the most promising results. Fisher was the principal investigator of a trial known as SANTE— Stimulation of the Anterior Nucleus of the Thalamus for Epilepsy. (*Sante* is the salute that the French give when they hold up their wine and toast to good health.)

SANTE was a two-year clinical trial at seventeen medical centers. It involved 110 patients. Doctors enrolled patients between eighteen and sixty-five years of age who had failed at least three antiepileptic drugs, meaning they continued to have at least six seizures a month despite the medicines they were taking. Sponsored by Medtronic, the study would determine if the medical equipment company—which had developed the technology that won government approval for use in Parkinson's, essential tremor, and dystonia—would get to market the device for intractable epilepsy. By July 2007, all the patients had been enrolled and implanted with stimulating electrodes.

One of those patients was Valori Kohler, a mother of two from Elwood Park, Illinois, who had her first seizure as a child. It was a rather odd effect. The seizure would spark a round of running. When she was in kindergarten she would bolt down the street, across Humboldt Park, and continue until her mother would catch her by the tail of her shirt and bring her to a screeching halt. It took years of running before doctors diagnosed the girl with complex partial seizures.

By the time Kohler was an adult, doctors had tried dozens of medicines. She would walk into a neighborhood grocery store, pick out something to purchase, put her money on the cashier's counter, turn on her heel, and take off running. Finally, she would fall on her face in a convulsion, wake up, and return to the store almost an hour later to complete her transaction. She had no memory of the time that she spent running, but people in her neighborhood knew that when Kohler came around anything was likely to happen.

As an adult, Kohler averaged five seizures a week and fell on her head hundreds of times. Medications made her look and feel drunk. There were brief periods in her life when the pills she took banished the seizures, but then they would return, or the side effects would overwhelm her and she would stop taking the drugs. Surgeons also tried vagus nerve stimulation, which failed to help her seizures at all.

Kohler had just turned fifty when neurosurgeon Roy Bakay of Rush University Medical Center in Chicago recommended a new experimental technique that might finally stop her constant seizures. Remember that Bakay worked at Emory with DeLong and Vitek; he moved to Chicago to become research director in the department of functional neurosurgery at Rush in 2000. Six years later, his patient, Kohler, was heading into surgery to have electrodes placed in her brain. Once the parameters of the stimulators were up and running, she began going days, then weeks, without an episode. She had about eight small seizures a month, and many of them stopped at the aura stage, with just a momentary strange feeling. Before the stimulators were in place, she would have thirty serious grand mal seizures a year. Now, she had one.

For Medtronic's device, called the Intercept Epilepsy Control System, to be federally approved, the company had to demonstrate a reduction in the rate of seizures in the three months after the stimulators were turned on. An independent safety monitoring group analyzed the results midway through the study to make sure that patients were not being harmed by the procedure. That the study wasn't stopped was a good sign that no harm was done; it also meant there was no increase in the number of patients' seizures. The company planned to announce the full study results by the end of 2008.

Stimulating inside the thalamus means that surgeons thread DBS leads all the way to the middle of the brain and into the central processing structure for every signal that enters the brain (except smell). It sounds scary, but in the hands of careful investigators and neurosurgical teams with highly precise methods of mapping their way to the target, the thalamus is building up a pretty good record as the go-to place to help patients whose lives have been altered by Parkinson's and other disorders.

The most common type of partial epilepsy in adults, however, originates in a less central place in the brain, the medial temporal lobe. Many patients with seizures originating in the temporal lobe that have not responded to medicines have found relief when part of the lobe was surgically removed. Now, with a new surgical tool on the block, the question was whether deep brain stimulation could work as successfully as cutting out a chunk of tissue did.

Kristl Vonck and his colleagues at Ghent University Hospital in Belgium had been pioneers in testing vagus nerve stimulation for epilepsy. In 2002, they recruited three epilepsy patients and used MRI and electrode mapping to make their way to an area called the amygdalohippocampal region. Once inside this tissue, they placed the electrodes to stimulate the focal, or originating, sites of the patients' seizures.

The team followed the three patients for five months; all had 50 to 90 percent fewer seizures.[38] It was perhaps more important that the patients' seizures were reduced without side effects, because as the region's name implies, the researchers were stimulating near two structures that have a great deal to do with how people understand who they are—the hippocampus, which processes memories, and the amygdala, which is a key structure in processing fear and other emotional experience, as well as being involved in human social interaction.

Meanwhile, back in Mexico, the Velasco brothers moved toward the temporal lobe with two studies that included a total of twenty-five patients. In the first study, with ten patients, they placed the electrodes near the amygdala and the hippocampus; in the second, they located regions in or near the hippocampus. Both were short studies lasting less than three weeks, except for three patients who remained with the stimulators turned on for three to four months. The brothers found significant reductions in most of the patients' seizures, and it was a benefit with no apparent side effects. Their younger patients had a more positive response to the stimulators than did older ones.

As part of the second study, the Velascos collected tissue samples to test the effects on brain chemicals within the region undergoing stimulation. Patients who showed the largest reduction in the number of seizures had high levels of a neurotransmitter called GABA, which dampens cell signaling. Those who didn't improve had high levels of benzodiazepine receptors. Such measurements might one day be used to predict which epilepsy patients might benefit from deep brain stimulation.

That improvements could be observed from stimulating either the thalamus or the temporal lobe is a familiar story in treating many disorders of the brain: some people benefit from a particular treatment, while others do better with something different.

Using electricity in the treatment of epilepsy is certainly not new. In the 1990s, transcranial magnetic stimulation—placing stimulating magnets on the skull to inhibit excitatory neurons on the topmost layers of the brain— became an option for patients. The concept had its root in Cooper's day, when King Coop stimulated the cerebellum. He placed his electrodes on the cortex. And in 2004 a group in Kyoto, Japan, reported reducing seizures in a single patient by doing the same procedure. But both Cooper and the Kyoto group had removed part of the skull to reach the brain's surface, while transcranial magnetic stimulation uses powerful magnetic fields to affect the brain's activity through the skull without surgery.

One company, NeuroPace, is developing a novel deep brain stimulation technique built with a microchip sensor, electrode, and microprocessor surgically embedded in the extracellular space within the brain to monitor abnormal electrical activity. Information of an impending seizure is sent to the microprocessor, which turns on the stimulating electrode to stop the seizure activity. The company calls this technology responsive stimulation. In 2008 NeuroPace was recruiting patients for a two-year clinical trial at twenty-seven locations around the United States to test the safety and effectiveness of the approach. The trials are slated to end in 2010. Other companies are developing similar technology.

In the studies of DBS with epilepsy, researchers noticed something that others doing follow-up on patients who had received deep brain stimulation for other disorders had also observed. Some patients had remained better than they had been before their surgery, even after the stimulators had been turned off. In 2000, the Velasco brothers noted a residual effect on their patients, whose seizures remained under control; however, after stimulation had been off for long enough, the seizures eventually returned to the presurgery levels. It could be that the stimulators actually reset abnormal connections—fixing the brain—or it's possible that a residual benefit from these devices lingers after the electricity has been turned off. Either way, it is proof that deep brain stimulation has a powerful benefit, though sometimes it comes at a hefty cost: side effects that occur in the normal course of tampering with the human brain.

Chapter 10

The Hardest Cases

Pain and Minimal Consciousness

You would think that as the first decade of the twenty-first century winds down, scientific progress on brain treatments would be rapid, and life would be getting better for patients afflicted with all but the rarest disorders. Even major forms of cancer now have good enough treatments that a remarkable number of people cope with it as a chronic illness rather than a death sentence. And heart disease is a growing success story as well, as people start to understand what cigarettes and high-fat diets can do to them.

Brain disorders, though, have been the new kid on the block when it comes to advances in medical research. The earliest attempt to draw the interior of the brain was in the seventeenth century, even though anatomy for the rest of the body was being documented in the eleventh century. And it took another two hundred years before physiologists could tell that particular diseases or behavioral events might reflect something going on with not the whole brain but just some part of it. Microscopes, chemical dyes, and other amazing research tools for looking at brain and nervous system tissue were developed in the twentieth century, but that century was almost over before ways of looking *into* the living and working brain were possible. It's really not surprising that progress in understanding and treating some profoundly distressing brain disorders—conditions about which almost everyone can tell a personal story—has been marked by deep frustration and achingly slow gain.

Two of the most heartbreaking conditions that have resisted the scientific exploration of the human brain are chronic pain and states of unconsciousness. While a walk down any drugstore aisle suggests plenty of ways to get at pain, neuroscientists have known for a long time that chronic pain will never have a drugstore solution unless they can figure out what triggers the abnormal brain signals that trip the sensory pain switch. And coma and other states of unconsciousness are a completely different animal. For centuries, if someone survived a loss of consciousness, he or she would eventually wake up or remain in that state indefinitely. Even scientists couldn't hope to understand the processes under way in the broken, unconscious brain.

These two brain states have something in common: scientists have had no way of measuring a person's experience. A patient with intractable pain can tell you that it hurts and even where it hurts, but there is no imaging device that can track down these pain signals and say, "Aha! *This* is what we need to do to stop the pain." As for states of unconsciousness, this is the Holy Grail of neuroscience. A patient in a coma or a persistent vegetative state can't voluntarily move or express himself, so there is no way to know what is going on inside him. Until recently, even peering into the unconscious brain yielded little information about how to turn the brain on so that its owner is aware of life around him.

To solve these problems, neuroscientists need the deductive imagination of Sherlock Holmes, the patience of Mother Teresa, and the optimism of the Wright brothers.

Neurosurgeon Ali Rezai, director of the Center for Neurological Restoration and staff neurosurgeon at Cleveland Clinic, has good measure of each of these traits. He was not the first to enter the field, but having studied with no fewer than five of the best neurosurgeons in the world, he knows the stuff neurosurgeons are made of, and he has become the unofficial spokesman in surgical scrubs for the field. As well, he knows that when national research budgets are pinched and innovative new treatments face multiple hurdles, a disorder or a line of research that has broad public support is likely to keep moving. When the media came calling after the first successes with deep brain stimulation, Rezai welcomed it. In 2007, President George Bush visited the Cleveland Clinic to hear more about medical innovations. He met with Rezai to learn about brain pacemaker technology and its application to movement disorders, and other emerging areas. An interactive presentation was provided during which President Bush performed a simulated delivery of a pacemaker electrode into a brain using brain navigation and delivery computer devices.

Rezai also made his department a hub of professional communication and collaboration with the top centers working on DBS and began organizing major conferences to bring together the pioneers in DBS research from around the world. His enthusiasm helped spread the word of the new technique and allowed scientists to develop and test novel ideas in the operating room.

In 1991, after finishing medical school at the University of Southern California, Rezai became a resident in the neurosurgery department at New York University School of Medicine. The department chairman was Joseph Ransohoff, a legendary neurosurgeon who had been in the same post since 1962 and was said to be the model for Ben Casey in the popular television series. Known to his coworkers as JR, Ransohoff was famous for hosting weekly meetings for his colleagues in neurosurgery to discuss vexing cases. JR exposed Rezai to the fundamentals of big brain surgeries—removing tumors, fixing aneurysms. After Ransohoff retired in 1992, his successor was Patrick Kelly, a major figure in the development of functional stereotactic surgery and a pioneer in computer-guided targeting and navigation in the brain. Kelly taught Rezai how to use computers to precisely and safely target various parts of the brain.

In 1996, Rezai accepted a fellowship at the University of Toronto to further specialize in the new field of functional neurosurgery. He started doing ablative surgeries and working with neurosurgeons such as Andres Lozano, to whom Helen Mayberg later suggested collaboration on DBS for intractable depression.

Rezai had broad neurosurgical interests—tumors, Parkinson's, psychiatric disorders, and brain injuries. DBS was a revelation—according to Rezai, "a defining moment in my life." Rezai recalled his first case, a patient in her sixties: "This woman was shaking for a decade; she couldn't button a shirt or drink a cup of coffee. But once that electrode was in place and the lead was stimulated, her arms were still."

In Toronto, Rezai also learned about the use of deep brain stimulation in treating unrelenting pain. His mentor was Ronald Tasker, who in 2005 would receive the Order of Canada, his nation's highest honor, and whose deepest research interest was treating pain. Tasker knew well how hard it was to engage clinical practitioners in new approaches to pain. In the 1980s, when he and other neurosurgeons were trying their hands at stimulating electrodes, Medtronic, the company supplying the leads, had become interested in pain as a possible target for deep brain stimulation surgery. The company had mounted a study on pain to test a new lead, but doctors were losing faith that it was working. Even in Tasker's hands, only half the patients improved—and they got only about 50 percent better. Unable to find enough surgeons for a clinical trial, Medtronic abandoned the studies.

Tasker had identified brain targets decades earlier by using microelectrode recordings of single cells as they responded to various painful stimuli. (Tasker's work aided Dr. Tipu Aziz, a distinguished neurosurgeon at the John Radcliffe Hospital in Oxford who helped launch DBS for unrelenting pain in the United Kindom. Aziz also used the technology to treat phantom limb pain, poststroke pain, and neuralgia.) Tasker, during his own training to become a neurosurgeon, had spent two years early in his career traveling through Europe to learn stereotactic neurosurgery. One of his mentors was Professor Lars Leksell of the Karolinska Institute in Stockholm, who developed radiosurgery, the still-used stereotactic frame, and surgical treatments for Parkinson's.

When Rezai's time was up in Toronto, he created his own traveling fellowship, a shorter one than Tasker's. He went to Grenoble for a few weeks to learn from Alim-Louis Benabid and then on to the Karolinska Institute before returning to New York University. "I picked up bits and pieces from a lot of surgeons and integrated the various pearls of wisdom from these experts into my own way of doing things," said Renzai. "There are different ways to skin a cat."

Back at NYU, ever eager to keep learning, Rezai continued working with Rodolfo Llinas, with whom he had trained as a research fellow for one year in 1993. The Llinas lab focused on using magnetoencephalography (MEG) and MRI to map the sensory and motor cortex and other brain functions. Llinas and colleagues established the role of the thalamus in regulating consciousness. His team demonstrated that the brain's electrical system oscillates, or vibrates, at a slower rate in the thalamus during sleep; the frequency of the electrical waves is much higher when awake.

Llinas and Rezai collected MEG recordings from the brains of patients with brain tumors, Parkinson's disease, epilepsy, and chronic pain and identified abnormal thalamic and cortical brain activity in these disorders. The thalamus filters sensory and all other cortical information. It serves as a gateway into the brain's cerebral cortex, the tissue that makes humans uniquely able to perceive, to think, to recognize, and to understand information from the environment at a high level.

Rezai was captivated by deep brain surgery and wanted to apply this new, reversible, adjustable brain pacemaker technology to other neurological and psychiatric disorders. The problem was that deep brain stimulation wasn't a priority in his department. The chairman, Kelly, was a tumor guru, so DBS would be no more than a part-time job for the NYU neurosurgical team. Economics was also a factor: DBS procedures were long, even by the standards of brain surgery; they were not reimbursed by insurance for the most part; and they required a lot of follow-up. Rezai left New York and headed for Cleveland Clinic to pursue his vision of developing the field of brain pacemakers.

Erwin Montgomery, Jr., now professor of neurology at the University of Wisconsin and a leading expert in movement disorders, established the deep brain stimulation program at Cleveland Clinic in 1997. Montgomery set up the recording system in the OR and worked with neurosurgeon Gene Barnett on patients with a variety of movement disorders. When Montgomery moved to Wisconsin in 2002, Rezai began to explore new ideas for Cleveland's program. He decided to use what he had learned about deep brain stimulation for pain during his fellowship with Tasker. One of the first patients he took into the Cleveland operating room was Megan Bruggeman, a twenty-five-year-old woman from Illinois who had been in unrelenting pain for ten years. But as Tasker had told Rezai when they had worked together a few years earlier, pain is a mystery that does not give up its secrets easily—not even under the weight of a technology like DBS.

Megan Bruggeman spent much of her childhood on her toes, spinning and moving gracefully. She wanted to be a prima ballerina when she grew up, but at fifteen she crushed a nerve. The injury triggered intense pain that wouldn't let up, and even after the nerve healed, simply stepping on her foot would send electrical jolts up her leg. Bruggeman tried just about everything to stop the pain—acupuncture, anti-inflammatory medicines, and a range of pain pills—but nothing worked. Ten years after her initial injury and still in debilitating pain, Bruggeman became one of the first people in the country to have electrodes placed into her motor cortex in an attempt to stop the pain message from getting through.

Rezai made a flap in Bruggeman's scalp, pulled it back, and removed a portion of her skull to reveal the outer layer of her brain. Then his team spent four hours stimulating virtually every area of her motor and sensory cortex to find the exact snippet of brain tissue that controlled movement and sensation in her left foot. Once they identified the target, they inserted a strip of four electrodes on the surface of the motor cortex and threaded wires beneath the skin of her scalp and neck, down to a tiny battery-powered device placed in her chest under her collarbone. Weeks after the stimulator was turned on, Bruggeman ran for the first time in years. She was able to concentrate and to sleep better. Her pain had dropped from a nine to a four on a scale of one to ten. The surgery took six hours, and she was awake the entire time, watching as they worked to identify the exact spot on the right side of the motor cortex that represented her left foot.

For four years, the motor cortex stimulator worked well for Bruggeman. Every six months, she would fly from her home in Chicago to Rezai's office at Cleveland Clinic for reprogramming. It would take multiple visits during these twice-yearly trips to get the device working just right. But then the programming stopped working. Rezai didn't know why. It became increasingly difficult to find an appropriate setting. Bruggeman's pain was back full throttle. She enrolled in new drug trials for pain, and none of the medicines helped. A year went by before Bruggeman and her mother, Nancy, frustrated and in despair, went back to Rezai. Rezai listened with compassion. Bruggeman had now been in pain for nearly two decades—most of her life. Rezai thought about the circuits of the brain, and then he suggested that maybe he needed to go deeper into the brain, into the thalamus. It took a year to get Bruggeman's insurance company to agree to pay for the procedure.

On January 7, 2008, Bruggeman went back into Rezai's operating room. Six months earlier, he had removed the leads on her motor cortex. This time, he would head for the thalamus on the right side of the brain. The thalamus is the brain's hub. It's like a relay station where information comes in and goes out. Calming this circuit might relieve Bruggeman of her pain.

With every neurological and psychiatric disorder, researchers believe, multiple regions may be effective targets for neuromodulation with DBS implants. Scientists now view the brain as a system with various networks implicated in different behaviors—everything from movement to cognition—and abnormal networks can be underactive or overactive. Scientists are still learning exactly how deep brain stimulation works to alter these networks—either by quieting some, as in Parkinson's, or by rousing others.

A day after the lead was placed in Bruggeman's thalamus, Rezai and his team met to talk about the programming. Could they get the right coverage to stop the aberrant pain signal? It was challenging. For years, her foot had been purple and black. It was hypersensitive and cold to the slightest touch. On the day Bruggeman arrived for programming, they played around with the settings until they found a particular frequency. With the device turned on, Bruggeman's leg turned bright pink and hot. Rezai was surprised. That Friday, they put everything together, attaching the electrodes to a new pacemaker-like device in her chest. The following day she was discharged to a local hotel. Two days later they set the parameters of the device, and mother and daughter flew home. Bruggeman's pain relief was dramatic—from a 9.5 down to a 3. "The pain story is a challenging one for all neurosurgeons," said Rezai, who was willing to try another region that he thought would help block pain signals. Bruggeman's experience was erratic, with some days better than others.

But over the next month her pain returned. To Rezai, the treatment had not failed; Bruggeman remained a work in progress. He would not give up trying to help his patient. "We need to be working harder at research to find the best target in the brain for pain," he said—his optimistic, Wright-brothers side in control.

Rezai's legacy may be either as a popular advocate for DBS technology or as the dogged neurosurgeon trying to make very sick people well with the technique. More likely to be forgotten is that he had something that all research enterprises need: the ability to make things happen. That talent was put to service when he helped to jump-start a study that would be the most dramatic in the short history of deep brain stimulation. The test would bring together a novel idea and the discovery that DBS stimulates the output of brain cells, and it would pit deep brain stimulation against the hardest challenge in all of medicine: consciousness.

In 1986, Nicholas Schiff, an undergraduate at Stanford University, received a scholarship from the Robert M. Golden Foundation to pore over the archives at the Montreal Neurological Institute. It had been ten years since Wilder Penfield had died, and only one Penfield seeker had ventured down to the archives, where dozens of pale green cardboard boxes were stacked on bookshelves. Inside the boxes were operating records scrawled with Penfield's notes, and for a young history and philosophy of science major in pursuit of the great old question—What is unconsciousness?—this was the fountainhead.

Schiff—everyone called him Niko—was heeding the message of a famous essay he had read by Gerald Holton, former head of the history of physics department at Harvard University: go back to the original idea, where the story begins. He had already read one of Penfield's classic works, *The Mystery of the Mind*, in which Penfield discusses his views on consciousness and how his studies on epilepsy patients helped him understand such states of altered arousal. And now Schiff sat in the archives and wiped the dust off Penfield's own files.

Among the things Schiff found were handwritten notes from Penfield to his friend Charles Hendel, a renowned Harvard philosophy chairman of the 1940s and 1950s who wrote an introduction to Penfield's book on the mysteries of the mind. The two friends studied the works of philosopher and psychological theorist William James, and in his notes to Hendel, Penfield discussed James's thoughts on consciousness.

Having gone to Montreal to study the philosophy of the mind and consciousness, Schiff was captivated by the writings. Then he met Theodore Rasmussen, a neurosurgeon who trained under Penfield and worked with him to define the motor homunculus. In 1950, Penfield and Rasmussen wrote what became a classic in the field of neuroscience: *The Cerebral Cortex of Man: A Clinical Study of Localization of Function*. Rasmussen took over for Penfield as director of the Montreal Neurological Institute in 1960, and it was said that he probably performed more epilepsy surgeries between 1955 and 1980 than anyone else in the world. In 1958, Rasmussen described a childhood condition in which a slow deterioration of one hemisphere of the brain leads to loss of function on the opposite side of the body. It became known as Rasmussen's syndrome or Rasmussen's encephalitis.

Rasmussen was seventy-six when Schiff knocked on his door at the Montreal Institute. Schiff remembered that Rasmussen's eyes were translucent blue and fixed on the young student as he listened to Schiff tell him about his project. The elder man then kindly interjected his view from the center of his universe: Penfield's classic theory of centrencephalic integration focused on how the thalamic intralaminar nuclei and related subcortical structures in the midbrain might bring together the functions of the two hemispheres of the brain and thus produce consciousness. The central thalamus plays an important role in the forebrain, Rasmussen told Schiff, and if you're thinking about consciousness, this is the place to start.

Rasmussen felt he was handing the young student the proverbial key to understanding issues of consciousness, but the science of the brain and the mind had shifted since Rasmussen's days as a prince of the field. The networks identified in the 1930s and 1940s were not getting much attention half a century later; research funding in the 1980s was going to scientists who were recording from single electrodes in the brain. While consciousness and arousal were fascinating topics at dinner parties, they couldn't sustain a modern laboratory.

When Schiff returned to Stanford to complete his senior year, he thought about something that Dr. William Feindel, curator of the Wilder Penfield archive, said to him before he left: "There are almost no neurologists left who are interested in consciousness." Feindel, a neurosurgeon who had shared the operating suite with Penfield and was a pioneer in his own right, had discovered the role of the amygdala in patients with temporal lobe seizures. "The only one is Fred Plum," Feindel said.

After Schiff completed his thesis on the role of the centrencephalic model and absence (petit mal) seizures in formulating Penfield's model of brain mechanisms underlying human consciousness, he began medical school at Weill Cornell Medical College in New York. On the opening day in 1987, at the traditional white coat ceremony for first-year medical students, he met Fred Plum, chairman of neurology. Excited, Schiff began talking Penfield and Montreal and consciousness. Plum smiled and told Schiff to stop by his office. It took three months of canceled appointments. "I'm a very busy man," Plum said when they met.

Plum had some simple advice: "Get your feet wet in research. You don't have much time. Science is a young man's game."

Plum knew from experience. In 1963, when he was thirty-nine, he went from being the only neurologist in Seattle to being chairman of the department at Weill Cornell. He succeeded Harold G. Wolff, who had founded the department and had served as its chairman since 1932. From his prestigious new position, Plum collaborated with Dr. Bryan Jennett, a Scottish spinal surgeon, to put the condition of persistent vegetative state on the medical map. They coined the term in 1972, and although many doctors had described these patients and even had attached names to this state, this was the one that stuck. "Persistent vegetative state" describes a person with a brain but with no knowledge, no language, and no awareness of life.

It is a rare phenomenon, Plum said, but modern medicine's life saving tricks were allowing the numbers of these patients to swell.

Patients in a persistent vegetative state look as if they are in a coma, but Plum and his colleagues uncovered the distinction between coma, which is a temporary state of unconsciousness, and persistent vegetative state. Patients in the first days and weeks of severe brain trauma are considered to be in a coma if they have no signs of a waking life; they remain with eyes closed and are unresponsive to stimuli and unable to be aroused. They may open their eyes in a few weeks but still be unresponsive. They seem to lack awareness. If they remain in this state for over a year, they will be taken out of the "coma" category and put into a group of patients described as being in a persistent vegetative state. The prospects for recovery are grim.

By studying these patients, who are normally sent away to languish in nursing homes, Plum's team began to see that some patients classified as persistently vegetative actually had some consciousness. Joseph Giacino, a neuropsychologist at the JFK Johnson Rehabilitation Center in New Jersey, and his colleagues developed criteria to describe such patients as in "minimally conscious" states. Thus, another name was born to define a different group of patients who were also cast off as too unresponsive for any type of modern-day therapies, including rehabilitation. These patients had some level of awareness, although as the name implies, it was minimal. They followed a voice on command, but only occasionally. Their awareness was fluctuating and fleeting, but there were moments when they uttered an appropriate word, made an intentional hand gesture, carried out some fitting action, or seemed aware of the environment and that they were a part of it. Plum put it this way: "The window shade is up for seconds or minutes and then goes down again."

Taking Plum's advice, Schiff plunged into research while still a medical student. He began working with Jonathan Victor, a brilliant Cornell neurologist who had entered Harvard when he was fourteen and was studying for a graduate degree in applied mathematics when other kids his age were packing up for college. Victor had gone on to medical school where, during his residency, Plum had spotted him and had decided the mathematician would make a terrific neurologist.

By the time Niko Schiff came along, Victor was an expert visual neuro-physiologist studying nonlinear dynamics in brain signals. Schiff's interest in the electrical workings of the brain was a good match. Schiff recorded the electrical activity of the brain during the moments when epilepsy patients lose awareness of their surroundings. It was a window into consciousness, and Victor shared Schiff's excitement about understanding the human mind. Working with Victor, first under a Howard Hughes fellowship and then during medical school, Schiff studied absence seizures. After Schiff's residency, Victor sponsored his first NIH career award, a grant that would allow Schiff to focus on how deep brain stimulation in the central thalamus affects visual processing. Schiff also began collaborating with Cornell's Keith Purpura, with whom he developed a detailed theory of the role of the central thalamus in visual awareness.

Schiff also joined Fred Plum in his laboratory. Plum's interest in persistent vegetative states led to the first brain scan studies in humans in these states. Plum had teamed up with Rodolfo Llinas at New York University; Llinas's tool was a noninvasive imaging technique, magnetoencephalography (MEG), which gives a relatively precise picture of electrical activity in the brain. Over the years, Llinas had used MEG with volunteers to study a range of cognitive functions, including how the brain processes silent meaning of a particular experience.

Llinas also had a long interest in consciousness, and he immediately signed on with Plum to study patients in a persistent vegetative state. In 1996, they brought their first patient into the scanner. Plum wanted to see what the machine would pick up from the brains of these patients, and Llinas wanted to know if their brains' electrical activity reached the forty-hertz activity of the waking, thinking brain. By that time, Schiff had earned his place on the team. From fall 1994 until 1997, Plum and Schiff went scouting for patients in a persistent vegetative state.

In 1997, Schiff submitted a patent application to use deep brain stimulation to improve the function of the human brain following stroke. At the time, he was thinking about people at a much higher cognitive level than those in a minimally conscious state (MCS). He was fascinated by patients who suffered from neglect syndrome, a condition in which patients no longer see a part of the body as their own or behave as if one side of the sensory space around them were nonexistent. Following a stroke or other trauma, some patients could easily follow commands from someone standing to one side—but not to the other. Schiff read a study about the use of cold water to stimulate arousal, and he tried it in patients with neglect syndrome. He took a syringe of ice-cold water and injected it into the right ear of a patient with a left-side neglect syndrome. She moved her left hand. "Whose hand is it?" he asked. "It's my hand," she replied. This recognition of half of her body was gone within three minutes. Schiff was hoping that deep brain stimulation could do what chilled water did.

Then Schiff met Cornell physician-ethicist Joseph Fins at a coffee shop at New York Hospital, a chance encounter that would change the trajectory of both their lives. Fins had been a visiting scholar at the Hastings Center in New York and was editing a column on ethics in medicine. Schiff told him about the collaboration with Fred Plum and Rodolfo Llinas, and Fins asked Schiff if he would like to write a commentary on a case that had just landed on his desk.

Fins had already carved out a niche in palliative care. It was an emerging field, and ethicists from all walks of life weighed in on pain management and end-of-life care. The patient in question for the commentary had end-stage cancer that had spread into his brain. He was in a coma. Should this patient be given pain medications? A resident on the unit said yes, but an attending physician argued that the patient couldn't feel pain, so why bother giving medicine to block pain? The question was: What could the brain perceive?

Plum, Llinas, Schiff, and their colleagues had already completed their first scanning studies of patients in a persistent vegetative state and had some evidence that parts of the brain were still active though not connected. They were ready to move on to patients in a minimally conscious state, but the funding establishment had minimal interest in them. Between 1998 and 2000, the team applied for four different federal grants to develop clinical studies on deep brain stimulation for patients in a minimally conscious state, and three were denied. The best they could do was a planning grant to get their ideas down on paper.

In 2001, the team finally received a grant to conduct another round of scanning, and this time it included functional magnetic resonance imaging studies, EEG studies, and PET scans. They collaborated with Joy Hirsch, director of the functional MRI laboratory at Memorial Sloan-Kettering Cancer Center. She had the tools, and she embraced the concept of using the scans to identify activity in the seemingly unaware brain.

That same year, the group brought two patients into the scanning device and played them taped narratives spoken by loved ones. Then they played the recordings backward, so that they were unintelligible. When the tapes were played normally, the patients' brains activated cerebral networks involved with the comprehension of language—the same region that would be active in normal, alert volunteers. When the tape was reversed, the same brain region was quiet. It was proof, the scientists believed, that at least these two minimally conscious patients understood the language of a loved one, and that the brain's language centers might be functioning on some level. The question was, How much and when? And would there ever be a way to increase the activity of their brains and allow more awareness to emerge?

Schiff and Fins, meanwhile, became fast friends and instant collaborators. Fins began shifting his focus from palliative care to consciousness, as he thought about such age-old questions as how much of your self you can lose before you are not you anymore. He saw the same kinds of patients that Schiff saw during his neurological rotations: patients who were not quite vegetative. They would respond on occasion, like a light that flickers, revealing something distinguishably human, but only for a moment. Imagine having awareness but knowing that you were being perceived as not there, Fins told Schiff. He knew what Schiff was up to in thinking about deep brain stimulation for neglect syndrome, but he wondered whether he really had the right patients in mind. Fins told his friend that if he was going to use stimulating electrodes to reconnect the broken brain, he'd better start with patients who had lost more than just recognition of half their bodies. Schiff knew Fins was proposing that he study minimally conscious patients, and he knew why: it would be easier to measure any benefit from the treatment. Fins also admitted it was a far-fetched idea; he was talking about patients who had been in a state of minimal consciousness for years, or even longer.

A short list of scientists had already tried to reawaken patients in various stages of impaired consciousness. In the late 1980s, Medtronic had set up a multicenter trial with neurosurgeons in Japan, France, and the United States to put stimulators into the right centromedial thalamus in patients considered to be in a persistent vegetative state. The investigators had implanted electrodes in almost fifty people. The work grew out of earlier reports from French scientists who had used deep brain stimulation in a handful of patients in a persistent vegetative state. A group of Japanese doctors also had found that electrical stimulation worked to bring some of these patients back to some level of awareness.

In 1990, as the last patients were being enrolled in the Medtronic study, one young woman who had been cleared for the study was flown on a special plane equipped for patients on life support from her Florida hospital bed to California. Terri Schiavo was twenty-six. Six months earlier, on February 25, 1990, she had collapsed in her home, where paramedics had found her unconscious and without a pulse. Her husband, Michael, had heard about the Medtronic study, and he hoped that deep brain stimulation could reawaken her. Surgeons in San Francisco had implanted an electrode into Schiavo's right centromedial thalamus, but the stimulators had done nothing to jar her back to consciousness, and the young patient had returned to Florida.

Almost a decade later, with no change in her status, Schiavo's case was at the center of a hotly debated issue on end-of-life care. In 1998, her husband went to court to allow doctors to discontinue life support on Schiavo. She was in a persistent vegetative state with no hope that things would change, he argued. Her parents fought the decision. In 2002, when Schiavo's brain scan circled the media globe, the Medtronic electrode was seen as a white spot on the right side of her brain. When she died in 2005, an autopsy revealed that the surgeons had hit the precise target. It just hadn't worked.

The study design had been flawed, and the results were disappointing. The selection of the patients, many of whom were in the first six months post-injury, when they might spontaneously get better, made it impossible to know the difference between a spontaneous recovery and a response brought on by electrical stimulation. It could be that the few patients who improved, all victims of traumatic brain injury, would have gotten better on their own over time.

Schiff examined the data from the Medtronic study and knew immediately that its concept was wrong. It was based on the earlier Japanese study, which had been designed without much attention to the nuances of vegetative states. To meet the criteria for the study, patients had no awareness of themselves or their environment, no response to sensory stimuli or comprehension of language or expression. They could have intermittent waking moments manifested by the presence of sleep-wake cycles. On all counts, Schiavo had fit the bill.

"They just thought that they could turn the electrodes on, and voilà!" Schiff said. "They didn't take into account the severity of the vegetative state and when it makes sense to put a stimulating electrode in to regulate function. It's not just sleep/wake that you want to change. You need an integrative brain."

Schiff approached Medtronic with a study designed after more than a decade of research, and the company offered Schiff's university a sum of $250,000. But it was a rather odd deal: the company wanted the patent rights but did not want to fund the trial. It had closed the chapter on consciousness and was working the more solid ground of movement disorders and, in time, psychiatric conditions. Cornell declined the Medtronic offer and looked elsewhere to find the money for the research.

In 2001, the team received almost half a million dollars in a federal three-year grant to develop a protocol to test deep brain stimulation for the treatment of patients in minimally conscious states. But the grant was allocated to design the protocol only; it explicitly stated that the group was not to use the money for clinical trials. By this time, Schiff had created a strong group of like-minded investigators willing to take on consciousness in these forgotten patients. Plum was in, and so was Schiff's mentor, Jonathan Victor. Joseph Fins was a definite. He knew just the right questions to ask as they moved forward in designing the studies. Joseph

Giacino, the neuropsychologist at the JFK Johnson Rehabilitation Center who had given the name to the minimally conscious state and had developed the criteria to define it, had worked with many MCS patients and had created the only rigorous and validated psychometric tool to measure outcomes in patients before and after deep brain stimulation. He was invaluable when it came to patient selection. To get an evaluation beyond bedside, the patient had to be able to have simple command-following abilities; gestures or verbal yes/no responses; some intelligible verbalizations; and movements or behaviors that were relevant to the environment. Neurosurgeon Ali Rezai, who had just returned to New York University School of Medicine, was also part of the study team.

It was Rezai's move to Cleveland Clinic that finally landed the team the money to try DBS on its first patient. The clinic's foundation had money left from a large grant from the State of Ohio, and Rezai was able to get it reassigned to the scientists to conduct the trial. For Nicholas Schiff, his passion to study consciousness was now fulfilled; they were headed into the operating room.

In the midst of the investigators efforts to identify the perfect first patient to test their hypothesis, a thirty-nine-year-old Arkansas man emerged from a minimally conscious state after almost twenty years. On July 11, 2003, Terry Wallis stunned his family by uttering his first word since suffering a severe head injury in a 1984 car crash. In the first months after the accident, the nineteen-year-old father-to-be had shown no signs of life beyond a beating heart and electrical activity in his brain, but his eyes would occasionally open, and sometimes he could follow simple commands to move his eyes toward an object, a sound, or a loved one. His close-knit family had visited the Stone County nursing home daily, never expecting that one day he would be asked by an aide, "Terry, who is this old woman who's come to see you?" and he would reply, "Mama."

During the first few weeks of Wallis's "awakening," his single words turned into sentences—short, meaningful, beautiful sentences that triggered an international media frenzy. Plum's team and others had run into the occasional patient who recovered function spontaneously after years of minimal consciousness. It was rare, but it happened.

127

By then, Schiff and his colleagues had already designed an experiment to implant stimulating electrodes into the brains of MCS patients with the hope that they could raise the shade and keep it up enough to let light—and life—in. The idea for the study had been ten years in the making—from identifying brain networks that shut down on the heels of brain injury to understanding which brain regions controlled these networks to finding the perfect test subjects.

The team believed that they now understood the damaged brain circuits that led to changes in behavior, cognition, movement, and neurological and psychiatric functions. They broke down each component and linked the damaged structure of the brain to functional changes in cognition, awareness, and behavior. Years earlier, Schiff had identified an area in the central lateral nucleus of the thalamus that acts as the gatekeeper to connect the brain's arousal centers to the basal ganglia, where other networks control cognition, language, and movement.

Now Terry Wallis's brain might be able to shed even more light on the subject of consciousness. Schiff called the doctors who took care of Wallis. His family agreed to allow the New York doctors, in collaboration with Joseph Giacino and his colleagues at JFK Johnson Rehabilitation Institute, to scan his brain on two separate occasions over a two-year period. They used many different scanning techniques, but the payoff came with diffusion tensor imaging, a way to measure the flow of water through the brain's white matter. They put Wallis through several lengthy batteries of psychological and cognitive testing to understand how he could suddenly awake from a nineteen-year state of minimal consciousness—talking and reacting, albeit much more slowly, as if time hadn't passed at all.

Henning Voss, an MRI physicist, analyzed the diffusion tensor imaging data. The brain scans showed something remarkable. It wasn't in the nature of an adult brain to grow new cells, but existing and even damaged cells could grow new connections. Wallis's brain had new neural connections around the extensive brain damage. As Wallis's weakened body got stronger—he could now move his limbs on command—the brain area controlling movement had grown even more connections. The brain growth was evidence that, as other research had been suggesting in recent years, the complex neural tissue was able to repair itself.

When Schiff stared at Wallis's brain scans, he saw something akin to an old house with new wiring. Some of the connections matched beautifully with Wallis's regained movement. His brain's metabolism provided scientists with the first glimpse of the possibilities that lay hidden in the damaged brain.

By the time the team published the brain changes in Terry Wallis, in the *Journal of Clinical Investigation*,[39] Schiff was director of the laboratory of cognitive neuromodulation at Weill Cornell. He and Giacino did all the surveying for DBS candidates. The first patient they selected had been part of the earlier brain imaging study by Schiff and Joy Hirsch. In October 2004, the team began a four-month-long series of tests to make sure the patient met all the criteria to be the first case for this landmark trial on deep brain stimulation.

The patient was a thirty-seven-year-old man who had been the victim of an assault and robbery six years earlier. His skull was crushed, and his brain had a large hematoma and massive swelling. After two months in a deep coma, he had emerged into the world with minimal alertness. He could open his eyes, and on the rare occasion he would utter a "yes" or "no" when asked a question. Mostly he was just silent, displaying a modest ability to attend to the environment around him. He met the medical criteria for MCS. Several brain scans done in 2001 showed that the regions necessary for language, cognition, and movement were spared from injury, just quiet. With research to guide them, the team knew where to put the electrodes and predicted how they might work to wake up the areas necessary to spark some recovery.

In 2005, the patient was flown from the JFK Johnson Center to Cleveland Clinic, where Ali Rezai was now heading up the neurosurgical deep brain stimulation program. The ten-hour operation was done in two stages. It was critical to make sure that the leads were implanted at the right location. After the surgery to implant the leads, the patient was taken for a brain scan to ensure that they had hit their mark. The stimulator was turned on for two hours following the surgery to make sure they had their target, but then kept off for the next fifty days of healing. The patient was back in New Jersey when the team turned on the device.

Within a few days, the patient was saying single words. In time, he was stringing together a few meaningful words at a time. To be assured that he was responding to the DBS and not to the surgery or the intense rehabilitation, the investigators carried out a six-month, blind crossover study. They turned the stimulator on for thirty days, then turned it off for the next thirty. Therapists who did not know whether the stimulators had been turned on or shut off measured the patient's ability to function. The cycle was repeated twice more.

The findings were clear. DBS had led to the patient's raised level of consciousness. Though he was still severely disabled, he regained some ability to speak and to feed himself. He smiled when interacting with family or staff, watched basketball on television, and expressed preferences. Almost a year after the implants were turned on for good, he recited sixteen words of the Pledge of Allegiance.

The team saw deep brain stimulation as a way to jump-start a minimally conscious brain to make it more active and to gain more functional recovery. Brain scans had shown that the network of cells in the thalamus that controls cognitive and motor regions was essentially offline— unavailable but not destroyed by the brain trauma. Targeting that area increased the overall activity of the brain regions that govern attention, arousal, communication, cognition, and responsiveness.

In the weeks after they published their results in *Nature*,[40] doctors involved in the study fielded calls from people who had loved ones lost to minimally conscious states. They wanted nothing more than the smiles and simple expressions of acknowledgment that the first study patient had managed. They saw interviews with his mother and wished for the day they could be in her shoes. "God bless the doctors who believed in my son," she had told the doctors who operated on her son. "My son, as well as the entire family, had little hope of further recovery. If it were not for the DBS surgery and rehabilitation, we would be no further along than we were in 1999. Now, my son can eat, express himself and let us know if he is in pain."

On one occasion, while many members of the team were visiting the patient at the rehabilitation facility, he seemed to be upset. "What's wrong?" someone asked him. "People," he said. "Too many people." Another time, he was stubborn and would not respond to his name. He finally told them that he had a nickname.

"Is your name Bill?" they asked.

"No."

"Is it something else?"

Without hesitation, he said, "Yes."

"His personality is slowly emerging," Rezai added. "He is very sweet." The mother said that before his accident he had enjoyed art and music.

It has been estimated that at least 100,000 patients throughout the country are living in states of minimal consciousness. With no evidence that treatment can help them, most have been put in nursing homes, forgotten by the world outside their families. But in his team's initial success, Schiff saw great hope. It led to plans to implant electrodes in another eleven patients. Cleveland Clinic started a medical device company called IntElect Medical, Inc., which raised millions to carry out the study.

The problem is that it is impossible to know who will benefit. Schiff and his team assessed hundreds of potential cases before landing on the few patients they ultimately would take into surgery.

The DBS researchers hoped their early results would change the way patients are treated following brain injuries. Meanwhile, the findings raised the bar on research. Steven Laureys, a physician with the Coma Science Group at the University of Liege in Belgium, had identified some subcortical activity in patients in vegetative states but had concluded that no high-level cortical network response was associated with the experience of feeling pain. "With functional imaging we can see what is happening in the pain matrix," Laureys said. "You see subcortical activity but it is disconnected from the regions that regulate conscious awareness." These areas are not disconnected in patients in minimally conscious states.

The Belgian scientist and his colleagues went on to scan seven vegetative patients five months after their injuries and asked them to imagine playing tennis or walking around their house. Two showed activity in regions of the brain that suggested they understood what the scientist said. Two months later, they both went from a diagnosis of vegetative to minimally conscious states. Laureys wondered whether the scanning technology gave scientists the opening to try to access whether someone will emerge from a vegetative state over time.

Adrian Owen, of the MRC Cognition and Brain Sciences Unit in the United Kingdom, developed functional magnetic resonance imaging scans to help identify residual stores of cognition in patients in persistent vegetative states and minimally conscious states. Owen and his team started looking for brain changes in response to sound perception, then speech and speech comprehension. Then they looked for signs of awareness. Could the patient respond to a command? They found that 40 percent of the vegetative patients had the same response to sound. The brains of three of the seven patients tested showed responses to speech itself. Normally, the brain makes a quick computation about what it thinks a person is saying. If it doesn't make sense, the brain reconfigures to make semantic sense of it. It's difficult to test comprehension of language itself, since 80 percent of words in English can be used in more than one context. Researchers are working on a test to do just that.

In the meantime, scientists have no idea what the DBS technology will ultimately mean for patients in states of minimal awareness. Awareness is a vexing state. Owen was treating a twenty-three-year-old woman who suffered severe axonal damage in a car accident. Axons are the long projections that allow information to travel from neuron to neuron, and damage to them can cause interference in the neuronal message trying to get through. Six months after the accident, the young woman was put into the category of persistent vegetative state. Owen and his colleagues used the same paradigm that Laureys had. The patient was put into a brain scanning device and was asked to imagine playing tennis, and the same region that is activated in normal volunteers responded to the request. Owen wrestled with solving this awareness problem. The patient's brain hadn't responded when she heard the word *tennis*, but when she had been asked to imagine playing the game, her brain had brightened. He was stumped.

Owen and his colleagues brought a dozen healthy volunteers in and put them to the test. As their brains were being scanned, the volunteers were asked if they had siblings; if they did, they were asked to imagine playing tennis. Then, if they had a female sibling, they were asked to imagine walking around the house, a response that should activate another discrete brain region. By asking just three questions, the scientists were able to show that normal volunteers can think of an activity as a way of answering a simple question. The scientists were able to answer the questions with 100 percent accuracy by just reading the scan, again suggesting that there are ways to tap into the brain of a person who is locked in and can't show signs of awareness.

"When we started doing this we never dreamed we could have a patient in a vegetative state imagining playing tennis," Owen said.

These studies, and the DBS-assisted reawakening of the assault victim who hadn't responded much in six years, raised a series of ethical questions about the treatment of patients in these altered states of consciousness. Perhaps most basic was the notion of reawakening patients to a more functional state, but one that is far from independent. "We need to look at the emotional aspects," said Schiff. "These are human beings, and we may be making people more cognizant of their own deficits. We can't ignore that." He and Fins began studying the ethical guidelines for deep brain stimulation research on this population of patients with a grant from the Charles A. Dana Foundation.

The Cornell/Cleveland/JFK collaboration also raised several issues about patients' rights: Does an unconscious patient feel pain? Can scans of the brain predict who will emerge from a minimally conscious state? Disorders of consciousness became the topic of the 2008 annual meeting of the Association for Research in Nervous and Mental Disease.

The new technology raises broader health policy questions: Should all head-injured victims have access to brain scans to find out if they can hear and understand and respond to commands? What is the medical obligation to pour resources into helping these patients strengthen or reawaken their broken circuits? And to what end? If it costs hundreds of thousands of dollars to enable one patient to sit up and eat on his own and respond on a simple level, is it an equitable expenditure of money and time?

The implications extend widely. Years of studies had led to understanding that DBS activated output through the axons of neurons at the site stimulation, and Niko Schiff has taken it a step farther. He proposes that activating output from critical regions of the thalamus with deep brain stimulation can activate or turn on areas of the brain that have not been integrated in years, or even decades. If he is right, then the federal government, insurance companies, and society will have to figure out what to do when a patient shows up at an emergency room unconscious and with a severe head injury. What therapies should be given? When should scans be done to see if some networks are still working but offline? And when should deep brain stimulation, or other future technology to reconnect the brain, become a viable treatment option in lieu of the standard custodial care?

The issues are highlighted by a comparison of two patients.

With team members monitoring his progress—and research money paying for it—the young man electrically stimulated out of his minimally conscious state by Schiff and his colleagues continued to receive physical and occupational therapy to enhance his recovery. He could sit up, answer questions, and have meaningful interaction with his family.

Terry Wallis was another story. Five years after his emergence, his mother was struggling to get him rehabilitation that would make him stronger, cognitively and physically. Insurance wouldn't pay for the treatment, despite the miracle of his reawakening. But Wallis wasn't complaining. He was home with his family, making his way in the conscious world. "Mama," he said, "life is good."

Part Three

Taking Stock and
Looking Ahead

Chapter 11

Patients, Parameters, and Risks

A s deep brain stimulation techniques have developed for each condition, the benefits always have emerged hand in hand with the side effects and the risks. In the years after the first federal approval for DBS, many centers began offering the surgery, and many did not have the expertise or experience to bring patients through the process successfully. There was a lot of enthusiasm for the technique, and sometimes it preceded the proof that the therapy would do more good than harm. "Some were moving way too fast without the ability to do it well," said neurologist Jerrold Vitek of Cleveland Clinic. Many of the leaders in the field were mentoring scores of people who went off to start their own deep brain stimulation programs.

Even the teams pioneering deep brain stimulation in their fields were seeing the numbers and their successes improve over time. The more cases, the more experience, and the better their patients were doing. But the failures from less-experienced groups, even neurosurgeons working solo, began showing up at the doors of better-known centers. The problem is that deep brain stimulation is not just a surgery but a technique that needs to be done just right—and, as we saw, sometimes adjusting the parameters of the stimulation can take months, or even longer. Then, as a disease progresses, as with Parkinson's, the device may need fine-tuning. And the batteries need attention; they must be tested routinely to make sure they are still charging the electrodes.

Chicago neurosurgeon Roy Bakay recently saw a patient who was having trouble with the stimulating electrodes in his head. They just weren't working to control his Parkinson's symptoms. Bakay had been in the deep brain stimulation business from the start, developing the DBS program with Vitek at Emory, and as a top neurosurgeon he was now seeing the failures of his colleagues who had not learned the trade well enough. The patient told Bakay that the neurosurgeon who had implanted the device was so happy with the surgical outcome, and the speed with which he had completed the procedure, that he had boasted, "I did it in two hours. I bet you won't find anyone who could have done it as quickly."

What took this neurosurgeon two hours to do was going to take Roy Bakay twenty hours to undo. The electrodes, it turned out, were in the wrong spot. "No wonder the patient didn't get better," said Bakay, who left his long tenure at Emory to oversee movement disorder surgery at St. Luke's in Chicago. "It was supposed to be the subthalamic nucleus on both sides of the brain. Neither one was positioned correctly."

Bakay, Kelly Foote of the University of Florida in Gainesville, and other experienced neurosurgeons were seeing a troubling and growing problem in the field. Medtronic had hired doctors and surgeons to sell deep brain stimulation through weekend seminars or at large medical meetings, and neurosurgeons who sat through the courses thought they could just go back to their operating rooms and try their hands at it. "They do a few and there are complications and they quit," Bakay said. "And that's when the patients show up at our door." The problems weren't easy to fix. "You don't even know whether they should have had surgery to begin with," Bakay said.

At Beth Israel Medical Center and then at Mount Sinai, nurse practitioner Joan Miravite became so proficient in programming stimulators—first to help surgeons reach their targets and then to find settings that would help control their patients' symptoms—that Medtronic ultimately hired her away. It was an indication of how critical the nonsurgical part of DBS is. Without proper programming, deep brain stimulation would not have survived. Few training programs are offered to health professionals, and a lot of programming is done by nurses, sometimes without physician oversight. "Most programmers have no idea about the anatomy or physiology of the brain," Vitek said. "Such knowledge would help immensely and would strengthen the success of individual programs."

There are four contacts on each electrode in DBS, and each contact does something different depending on where in the brain it has been placed. Even a millimeter along the lead is significant when it comes to brain tissue. In Parkinson's, certain contacts are better for dyskinesia, and others influence tremor.

When DBS is used to treat depression or OCD, a psychiatrist needs to drive the programming because both the benefits and the side effects are emotional and behavioral. So, for example, Cleveland psychiatrist Donald Malone screened every patient who walked through the door as a candidate for the experimental surgery, and he conducted all intraoperative stimulation and the programming that followed. Malone has probably programmed more patients with obsessive-compulsive disorder and depression than anyone in the country. He followed thirteen patients— five with obsessive-compulsive disorder and eight with depression—for at least six months and reported that almost half were doing better.

Malone followed the standard procedure of beginning with one contact and testing the functional response to it, then moving on to the next. At each contact, he changed the voltage, as well as the amplitude of the pulse and its frequency or duration. Because each patient responds differently, it can take three to six months to find a good setting for Parkinson's disease and much longer for psychiatric conditions.

Some contacts, when stimulated, brought on anxiety, sweating, warmth, or sadness. At each contact, Malone wrote down the response, titrated the frequency and amplitude, and jotted down some more notes. On some contacts, patients experienced an elevated, almost manic mood, and he lowered the settings. It was hard work getting them right. The initial programming took hours over a three- to four-day period. After ninety minutes, patients were so tired that they needed a break before continuing with several more hours of programming. Then they returned the next day for the same slow torture of stimulating and describing every thought or behavior.

Rob Weil, the physician in Hershey, Pennsylvania, with dystonia, called Joan Miravite whenever he sensed trouble. A few weeks after his DBS surgery and before the programming was set to begin, his arching movements stopped on their own. Weil imagined that the globus pallidus was shocked by the surgical procedure and had stopped sending out its abnormal signals. Two weeks after his miraculous respite, his symptoms reemerged full throttle.

The programming team had to wait three more weeks for the swelling in his brain to subside. When it was time to have the device turned on, the programmer started with the lowest voltage and worked his way up. At the time, many in the deep brain stimulation world thought more was better. They would learn that this just wasn't so.

Even after Weil had two leads replaced and another round of repro-gamming, the ultimate setting was altered until his programming got it right. In the end, the original pulse width of 400 was reduced to 270. The frequency of 130 dropped to 100, and the 3.1 voltage setting was turned down to 2.5. With the right settings in place, the abnormal movements that had wracked his body since medical school were virtually gone. And when he needed a scan that required turning off his device, he took his "professional hand-holder," Miravite, with him. If it was off for more than a minute or two, his symptoms returned and it took another two weeks to calm his neck muscles. Everything was timing.

DBS can present other problems as well. The leads can be put in the wrong place, or they can fracture; the extension that goes from the lead to the battery pack can erode or break; and the implanted pulse genera-tion can malfunction. Hardware troubles seem to occur in anywhere from 10 to 30 percent of DBS patients. These problems can be managed with routine visits to the DBS team, but patients must also be aware that the batteries run out without warning, which can trigger symptoms. Devices have been known to turn off when they encounter some types of electrical interference. Patients can no longer undergo certain types of scans and must remember to alert airport security about the device. Medtronic also put out warnings about using diathermy, a procedure used for the treatment of pain or inflammation. The device heats tissue. There have been several reports of DBS patients using diathermy who suffered heating at the site of the stimulation electrode interface. This can cause permanent tissue or nerve damage.

There is no doubt that deep brain stimulation changed Mario Della Grotta's life dramatically and for the better. His checking and obsessing dropped from fourteen hours a day to four. He went back to school and was raising two children with his wife. But it was also true that his brain was now intimately tied to an artificial electrical circuit that could weaken without warning and leave him vulnerable to a new set of problems. A dying battery had led to his ordeal with the state trooper. It wasn't just his obsessive counting that came back with a vengeance that evening on the way to the hospital. He also made an impulsive decision to flee the scene without giving thought to the possible consequences of his actions.

As the use of DBS caught on, such situations became the concern of professionals such as Laurence Tancredi, a psychiatrist and lawyer in New York, who wondered whether electrical stimulation could have a spreading effect on brain networks and result in unforeseen problems. In Della Grotta's case, it may have spilled over into judgment issues. "His broader cognitive issues may have been affected," Tancredi said. It's possible that Della Grotta's reemerging symptoms could have been prevented had there been a way to know that his battery was low or, in the case of other patients, that the device wasn't working properly. A device is no different from a medical treatment. It may not work, and it comes with side effects. (Medtronic and other companies emerging on the DBS front are working on the next generation of devices, including better electrodes and wiring and smaller, more powerful batteries with computer chips that could alert the patient to any malfunction in the device.)

University of Florida neurologist Michael Okun and his DBS partner, neurosurgeon Kelly Foote, were having a run of "redos" from other doctors. They saw so many that they became the authorities on side effects and other problems that emerged from the deep brain stimulation world. They, along with Alterman and Tagliati's team at Mount Sinai, saw a total of forty-one patients who walked in after someone else performed the surgery. Half the surgeries had been done improperly. The other half of the patients had problems that could be solved with proper programming and/or medication adjustments. In all cases, the problem was a lack of expertise by the original doctors.

Selecting the right candidate for deep brain stimulation is not easy. In the best of cases it is a team effort with surgeons, neurologists, psychologists, and other professionals who know the technology. Even if patients walk in with all the signs of Parkinson's disease, about 20 percent of them may have another movement disorder that looks and feels like Parkinson's but isn't. And if the DBS device is implanted in these patients, they could be worse off than before.

Michael Okun fell in love with the brain in medical school. He was so fascinated by people with wild, uncontrolled movements that during a neurology residency at the University of Florida in 1996 he carried around a video camera and taped patients in all sorts of physical perturbations. He got particularly hooked on the basal ganglia movement disorders. He was also working in a huge clinic at the nearby VA hospital, and during his first few weeks there he met a wheelchair-bound young man with Parkinson's disease. Johnny had such severe on-and-off fluctuations that he had been unable to walk for years. Without any supervision—neither of his institutions had a formal movement disorders program—Okun hit the books and tried any number of things to help his patient. Finally, he videotaped Johnny when the medication worked, then when it worked too well and he was having spontaneous flailing movements. Such dyskinesia is a common side effect of L-dopa therapy.

Okun sent the video footage with a long medical note, including the man's history, to Philip Starr, a surgeon at the University of San Francisco. Starr had done a clinical fellowship in microelectrode-guided surgery at Emory. He was interested in the physiology of the basal ganglia and was at the forefront of deep brain stimulation for Parkinson's and dystonia. His mentor was Roy Bakay.

Okun had read about Starr and a study he was conducting on the DBS technique for Parkinson's, which in 1998 was hitting its experimental stride. Okun thought the videotape would help get Johnny into the study, and he was right. Starr agreed to evaluate Johnny, and Okun negotiated with the VA system to buy him a round-trip ticket from Florida to California. Starr performed the surgery, and his team programmed the electrodes and sent Johnny back to Florida. "I remember the absolute awe in seeing him in the clinic without a wheelchair. There were no fluctuations and he was just walking. I remember looking at him, thinking, 'My God. I am not sure what they did but it is pretty amazing.'"

That was the defining point in Okun's career. The surgery was so successful that the young patient was preaching from the rooftop; he threw away the wheelchair and walked without assistance for the first time in years. Starr said he was one of the most dramatic cases he had seen. Had Johnny emerged from the surgery in any other form, Okun might have taken his career in another direction. But the results convinced him he had found his calling.

Okun looked for a fellowship in which he could get into the operating room with the surgeons and place deep brain stimulators. Like Starr, he found one at Emory. During his second year, with Jerrold Vitek as his mentor, he learned how to do microelectrode recordings during surgery. He was so excited that he would sometimes send one of his videotapes highlighting a unique patient to Philip Starr or to other movement disorder experts.

"Every once in a while things line up perfectly," Okun said. "I was like a kid at a carnival."

Okun was hungry to see patients, and over time the videotapes allowed him to catch what some of his colleagues failed to see in their practices: complications. He began collecting these problems piecemeal from many movement disorders clinics. Together, his collection made a large and important series. His first major paper was published in the *Archives of Neurology* in 2001, and it received a color photograph on the cover.[41] Okun was still on his fellowship, and he learned a lesson that would inform the next chapter of his life.

In neurosurgery, history is a critical piece of the puzzle. In 2002, Okun returned to establish a movement disorders program at the University of Florida in Gainesville. By then, he had learned that the only way to know the benefits and the risks of deep brain stimulation was to ask a lot of questions of the patients who were returning to the clinic with problems and to understand the backstories of the events in their lives before and after the surgery.

His time in the operating room at Emory had helped Okun think like a neurosurgeon. In accepting the challenge of founding a movement disorders program and bringing deep brain stimulation to Gainesville, he knew that it wasn't enough just to *think* like a brain surgeon. He needed one on his team. He found Kelly Foote.

Foote spent his undergraduate years studying engineering, and so tinkering was a way of life for him when he signed on to medical school. He wanted to be a neurosurgeon, and he accepted a residency at the University of Florida, where he learned about computer-guided neurosurgery. He went on to a fellowship with William Friedman, a neurosurgeon who, with nuclear engineer Frank Bova, developed a surgical system used around the world. From there, Foote went to France to work with Benabid and, returning stateside, spent a short stint doing deep brain stimulation with Mahlon DeLong and Jerry Vitek at Emory.

When Foote and Okun teamed up to start drawing on the blank slate of the new movement disorders program at the University of Florida, both had training in neurology and neurosurgery, and they thought hard about what was needed to develop the deep brain stimulation program and to seal the treatment's place in medicine. Drawing on Foote's background in engineering and Okun's penchant for history (it was his undergraduate major), they set up a computer database that would allow them to collect information about each patient, from the start of the selection process to the surgery and on into years of visits to the center.

Most of the 40,000 patients who have had deep brain stimulation are Parkinson's disease patients. For them, an initial workup was critical to rule out any other movement problem that would not benefit from the treatment. With that piece of the puzzle out of the way, the team had to assess the patient's cognitive status. Any history of cognitive problems or untreated depression or mood disturbance could recur or worsen following surgery. Also, the risk of a brain bleed is greater in older patients and in those with high blood pressure. And neurologists considering deep brain stimulation for a Parkinson's patient must make sure that the patient has a documented response to L-dopa. DBS works by reducing the same symptoms that respond to L-dopa, so patients who don't have that history are poor candidates for the surgical technique.

The extensive database allowed Foote and Okun to get a clear picture of the post-DBS infection rate. Okun found that, in the best of hands, about 6 percent of patients would suffer an infection, and more than half of those would do well with an antibiotic. Patients who developed pus around the site of the device faced a serious infection and needed immediate treatment. Since 2002, the Florida group had removed the electrodes and the batteries from many DBS patients who developed infections. And some of these patients' DBS surgery had been performed by teams that knew what they were doing. It is a surgical risk that, for most patients, is worth the benefit.

It wasn't always easy to identify infections once the patient left the hospital, returned for programming, and was reaping the benefits of the treatment. Foote's worst DBS experience was with a man in his early sixties with Parkinson's whose body was very brittle. Before deep brain stimulation, he spent his entire day frozen or making uncontrolled dance-like movements; he wore a seat belt to stay secure in his wheelchair. When strangers saw the man, they were convinced he was having a seizure. He could not move at all when his Parkinson's medication wore off, and this had been going on for more than three years. Deep brain stimulation ended it; his wild movements were gone, as was his wheelchair.

Before the surgery, Foote had his usual talk with the patient about side effects to watch out for. In the Florida group, there was a 5 percent chance of infection, and he told the man that about half of patients who developed infection would have it severely enough that the device would have to be taken out. But when swelling and redness appeared around the patient's scalp incision, the man put on a baseball cap to hide it. When pus oozed out, he didn't tell anyone. He loved walking and moving about without freezing; no way was anyone going to take the device out and land him back in his wheelchair.

The infection won out. Paramedics took him to the emergency room in a coma and with a huge abscess in his brain. Foote removed the device, and the patient was in critical condition in the intensive care unit for three weeks. After another two months in the hospital, he continued to recover, but his Parkinson's symptoms were back to where they were before DBS surgery. "When can I have surgery again?" he asked Foote. The question was familiar to doctors with experience implanting deep brain stimulators; some patients said they would rather die than go back to shaking and freezing.

Foote agreed to reoperate, but he told his patient he'd better not try to beat an infection again. The second surgery was a success, and he escaped infection, but he would never forget how close he came to dying. The two biggest factors in reducing the chances of side effects are the doctors and the patient—matching a medical team with a lot of experience in DBS with the right candidate for the treatment.

"It is a lot of work to manage these patients," said Okun, who is also interested in why deep brain stimulation does not always return people to work. "It turns out to be a complex issue, and the promise of stimulation has not always translated into helping people move back into the workforce."

Okun's team also began noticing that many of the patients showing up at their door were not good candidates for surgery. If a patient had cognitive problems before surgery, it could well tip the scales when a part of the brain received stimulation to stop motor movements. It was becoming clear that many surgeons were embarking on deep brain stimulation without a real understanding of what should go right and what could go wrong. Often it was a matter of poor programming and follow-up.

Before Okun left Emory, Vitek had helped him write an NIH grant to study mood and cognitive changes in Parkinson's patients following deep brain stimulation, and he was able to bring this funding to Florida. When Okun and Foote began studying patients, they would identify the contact that was used to control their tremors and rigidity and then stimulate it to look for any cognitive or behavior changes. Then they added a new set of DBS patients to their analysis—those with OCD, Tourette, and other disorders. One of the first things they noticed was that when stimulated in specific regions people smiled, laughed, or cried, and these behaviors had no relationship to their mood. They would look at all sorts of behavior and mood changes on and off stimulation and in different locations than those traditionally tested, and they began to see patterns. They asked questions that others may not have thought to ask.

Okun and his team also began comparing the neuropsychological changes before and after deep brain stimulation in Parkinson's patients who had electrodes placed in the globus pallidus or the subthalamic nucleus. The Florida DBS specialists looked at the effect of DBS on memory, concentration, apathy, and motivation.

"Deep brain stimulation operating rooms and clinics are the ultimate living human laboratory," Okun said. "I saw things and began to appreciate that these were side effects, and potentially benefits, of the technique and these may be utilized for targeting and tailoring specific symptoms and disorders."

Okun and Foote began publishing these and other results (smiling, crying, laughing, anxiety, panic attacks), and doctors started referring patients who were having problems or not getting relief from the treatment. Entering the data from these patients into the system, Foote and Okun realized that many of their colleagues were not screening properly for the right patient. They wrote and published a triage screening tool called the FLASQ-PD in the journal *Neurology*, and they began to advocate strongly for complete multidisciplinary screening for DBS patients. Later, Okun would carry this multidisciplinary and interdisciplinary approach to patients with him when he was appointed national medical director of the National Parkinson Foundation. He learned an important lesson: if the surgeon didn't have a whole team of specialists (neurologists, neurosurgeons, psychologists, psychiatrists, physical/occupational therapists, and speech therapists) working to identify the right patients, the wrong patients would get through. Okun and Ruth Hagestuen at the

National Parkinson Foundation joined forces to advocate for this approach for all Parkinson's disease and movement disorder patients.

In 2004, Okun, Foote, and Wayne Goodman, a psychiatrist at the University of Florida who was an expert in obsessive-compulsive disorder, landed the first NIH grant for DBS in OCD. They collaborated with their colleagues at Brown and Cleveland Clinic, as well as Bart Nuttin in Belgium, to make intraoperative observations of one-sided smiles induced by deep brain stimulation in a patient with obsessive-compulsive disorder. The patient had electrodes placed in the right and left anterior limb of the internal capsule and in the nucleus accumbens. During the surgery, they observed changes in facial movement during stimulation. The surgery was recorded. Okun had invited neuropsychologist Dawn Bowers to the operating room that day because she had been doing important work involving recording light reflectance patterns on the faces of Parkinson's patients to measure expression. In a true case of being in the right place at the right time, Okun, Bowers, and a graduate student named Utaka Springer captured, measured, and proved this abnormal one-sided smile response. Benjamin Greenberg, Steven Rasmussen, and their colleagues at Brown were actually the first to identify this odd upper turn of the mouth. The field initially criticized and rejected the finding, but the team persisted in publishing their results. The Brown group's initial observation was also published.

The abnormal facial grimace is now something to look out for in DBS procedures. The teams had observed that when the electrode was turned on, the patient consistently developed a half smile on the opposite side of the face. The half smile disappeared when the device was turned off. And they reported something else: when the nucleus accumbens region was stimulated, the patient reported feeling euphoric. (The accumbens is the brain's reward center.)

Okun and Foote continued taking careful notes about what worked, what didn't, and what patients could expect in the way of benefits and side effects. In addition to the half smile, they found that patients sometimes experienced funny smells and unusual tastes when the stimulator was on. They could experience happiness or anxiety. Even panic attacks could be triggered by too much stimulation at a certain contact. The researchers also had their share of misadventures. One time a patient with obsessive-compulsive disorder was reported missing after he had been discharged from the hospital following DBS surgery. The fifty-year-old man was finally found in the parking lot of the hospital twelve hours later. His symptoms were so strong that he could not get himself to turn on the car and drive home.

Keeping pace with the increased use of deep brain stimulation was a growing list of side effects that Okun, Foote, and other experienced surgeons were describing after years of operating on, programming, and following up on patients. Emerging were subtle problems with memory, cognition, apathy, and motivation that could well be triggered by the spread of electrical signals from the stimulation site to the brain's associative and limbic regions, which govern thoughts and mood. Some patients also developed speech problems.

One such patient was neurosurgeon Ali Rezai's third case, Richard Kramer, a social worker who had been diagnosed with Parkinson's at age thirty-six. Although it was a price Kramer was willing to pay to get his body back, he lost the fluency of his speech to deep brain stimulation. The young man had improved so much in the first month after the surgery that he was able to play tennis with his surgeon, but during the rest of his first year, he returned almost thirty times to New York University Medical Center for help in easing his speech problems.

One of the most vexing problems for Kramer was that people could no longer understand what he was saying. Words ran out of his mouth so fast and so low that the syllables melted into one another and made no sense to anyone listening. In time, doctors realized that some patients with leads implanted bilaterally into the subthalamic nucleus suffered from these speech problems, and no readjustment of the parameters would make words come out any better. Kramer experienced another problem: he went into surgery without a tremor but emerged with one.

As for the surgical redos showing up around the country, some centers were telling these patients to go back to the center that had implanted their devices. But Okun, Foote, and neurologists Hubert Fernandez and

Ramon Rodriguez, also in Florida, embraced the opportunity to care for the patients and to learn as much as they could about the more subtle side effects of the technique. They applied what they had learned about true interdisciplinary care. When a redo walked into their office, they invited the patient to come for an extensive two-day evaluation. They rated the patient on a series of clinical scales in all conditions (with and without medicines and with DBS on or off), obtained an MRI scan, and measured the locations of the leads. Then they would program the device to find the right threshold for benefits and side effects. As of 2008, they had brought nearly two dozen patients back to the operating room to put the electrodes in the right spot. And they documented everything they saw along the way in an effort to help the field move forward. Okun, always the fan of history, preached to his students to "keep your eyes wide open and look for the data and beware of dogma. You can help people even when you may initially think you can't."

The team's database helped inform the field, and they became crusaders in the fight to ensure that every patient has a complete neuropsychiatric screening before being accepted as a candidate for DBS. All of the major centers testing deep brain stimulation were doing presurgical neuropsychological evaluations; only after the technique began spreading to other centers did they find patients being accepted into surgery without such detailed assessments.

As Okun and Foote saw it, the problem was the lack of consensus on who should qualify for the procedure. Without a standardized reporting system for adverse events, it was not clear what would turn up years down the road.

Okun and his colleagues continue to develop patient selection standards for all the conditions now targeted for deep brain stimulation. He is hopeful about the possibilities once standards are in place.

Chapter 12

Ethics and the Future

Working with psychiatric conditions has added a new layer in problem solving as deep brain stimulation finds new uses. Many movement disorders take weeks or months of programming to find the right parameters, and even with the exact settings, it just takes time for the brain to respond. It may be harder for psychiatric patients to take a wait-and-see attitude. DBS teams have to make sure these patients understand that they will continue to have symptoms. And the procedure might not even work. Some early results on DBS for obsessive-compulsive disorder and depression show that it may work to some extent in around 50 percent of patients. But given the fact that nothing else has made a dent in the patients' symptoms, this may be a surgical risk worth taking.

Psychiatric patients pose other ethical problems as well. Patients for whom nothing else has worked often have a history of suicidal thoughts or behavior. Brown's Benjamin Greenberg stopped keeping a waiting list for patients with depression or OCD after a patient on the waiting list killed himself. Another young man threatened to kill himself if he did not get into the study. The team grappled with these issues during long ethical debates. How do you find a patient who will not be a threat to himself or to the study? If these patients are the worst cases, then high risk is already built into the equation.

Risk and tragedy had even touched the first small pilot study using deep brain stimulators in the United States. The study was carried out in 2003 at the University of Michigan, which had received federal and local approval to place electrodes into five patients with OCD. One of these patients ended her life more than a year after having electrodes implanted. DBS had given her a great deal of relief from her obsessive symptoms, but it had not helped the severe depression that also tormented her. A few days before her death, she wrote a letter to her doctors at the university and arranged for it to be delivered to them after she was gone. She wanted her doctors and the wider world to know that the device was working fine. She said that her decision to end her life had nothing to do with the treatment. She was only the second psychiatric patient treated with DBS at Michigan. Even as she made plans to end her life, she wanted to protect the technology and its ongoing development.

"My suicide is in no way connected to or a result of Deep Brain Stimulation," the patient wrote. "DBS relieved many of my OCD symptoms," she continued. "My DBS gave me the ability to function nearly independently if it were not for depression. OCD no longer became a major factor in my life after the surgery. Suicide was a choice I made now, but tried and thought about long before the surgery. DBS will save many people from OCD and its terrors. I couldn't save myself now because of so many dimensions of depression and instability that I have lived with for years. ... DBS surgery should not be stopped. It will save many lives."

The patient's death occurred just over fourteen months after her implant surgery. She had decided to continue the treatment because she found it so helpful for her OCD, but those benefits were not sufficient to save her life. She was one of the first OCD patients to receive DBS. With time and growing experience, the best target within the brain has shifted slightly. The use of DBS for depression may have helped her—but these studies were not yet available when she took her life.

In 2004, Andres Lozano and his colleagues from the University of

Toronto reported the results of a study on suicide risk in Parkinson's patients who had undergone subthalamic stimulation. They surveyed sixteen surgical centers, and half of them responded, with information on more than 400 patients. There were two suicides and seven attempts. When they scanned the published studies on deep brain stimulation, they found four attempts and two suicides in 153 patients. The suicides had occurred within three months to three years of the surgery, while the attempts had happened within five years of the implantation. At that same meeting, another team of doctors counted six suicides in 140 DBS patients within seven years of their surgery. Four of these patients had a presurgical history of depression.

In the world of refractory depression, these numbers are much lower than would be expected. There is evidence that without the proper treatment, 15 percent of these patients would have ended their lives. Psychiatrists working with DBS patients are constantly monitoring them for severe depression and suicide risk and readjusting the stimulating electrodes in the brain to help bring about relief.

In the best of DBS hands, an ethicist has always been part of the team. Raymond DeVries, a professor of bioethics at the University of Michigan Medical School, worked on a consent form for a study using deep brain stimulation for patients with severe treatment-resistant depression. He wanted to make sure the form would make clear that the procedure they would undergo was not a therapy but a surgical study to answer questions about whether DBS *could* be a therapy for patients who had not responded to any other available treatment. "We don't want people on the study team to give patients false hope," DeVries explained. "But clearly there is an expectation that the technique works and that they may get better."

The ethicist must consider whether a patient volunteer has the cognitive ability to understand the procedure and the risks it carries. An ethicist is also important when something unexpected arises around informed consent.

Paul Ford is a bioethicist at Cleveland Clinic. He was called down to evaluate a Parkinson's patient on the operating table who was almost to the end of surgery when he wanted to stop. His anxiety had gotten the better of him, and he wanted the surgeon to stop what he was doing and sew him up. He had been through all the risks of surgery already. He was mildly sedated but awake, and the team wanted to know whether they were ethically obliged to march forward and finish the surgery or stop. Ford met with the neuropsychologist. He then went to speak to the family. The patient's family said that the patient did tend to get extremely anxious, but he expected that even during these states people would listen and respond to his wishes. At that, Ford spoke with the surgical team and they sewed the man up. Two weeks later, the patient called the surgeon and said he was ready to reschedule surgery. The surgeon said no. They didn't think that the risk of another round of surgery was worth the benefit, especially if he should get anxious and change his mind again.

The ethical issues get even more complicated when psychiatric patients are involved. Several studies are under way to figure out whether deep brain stimulation really works for OCD and depression. To truly assess the treatment, there is a so-called sham period, when the device is turned off without the patient's or the doctor's knowledge. (The patient remains on whatever medications or therapies he was on prior to the surgery.) During this time, patients are asked to keep detailed records of their moods, behavior, and thoughts. It can be an arduous task for patients in the throes of a deep and lasting depression, but it's the only way to carry out a rigorous scientific study. The companies developing these devices for psychiatric conditions need the information to make a case to the Food and Drug Administration. If the FDA approves the device for a certain condition, insurance companies will generally pick up the bill.

As you may now realize, a good DBS team includes a neurosurgeon, a neurologist, a psychiatrist, a psychologist, and an ethicist. The ethicist helps inform the design of the study and, in many cases, is involved with talking to patients about the experimental procedure and making sure that they understand that it is not a tested treatment. While it is implicit that the technique might have a benefit, no one can ever promise that it will alleviate suffering. The patients who want to take part in these experimental surgical studies have tried and failed dozens of treatments. They arrive at the door desperate.

It is this desperation that scares DBS teams. In the best of teams, everyone meets with potential patients to ensure that they can withstand not only the surgery but also the aftermath of programming and follow-up.

In 2003, on the verge of his work with deep brain stimulation to awaken the brains of patients in minimally conscious states, Joseph Fins wrote in *Neurology Clinics of North America* that "any student of medical history would have to ask if these developments are ethically appropriate and whether the promise of neuromodulation will be able to transcend the potential peril associated with manipulation of motor, psychiatric or cognitive functions."

Mario Della Grotta would say yes, deep brain stimulation was worth it—even when his batteries wore out. His life was no longer swallowed up by counting and washing and the compulsions that took over most of his pre-DBS days. For Melissa Murphy, her depression had lifted enough that she no longer had days when she hid under her covers to escape the world. For the first time in years, she saw the possibilities in a day.

But the concerns voiced by Fins and others become louder as DBS spreads as a treatment for more kinds of conditions. In 2003, University of Toronto neurosurgeon Andres Lozano took a 420-pound man into the operating room to implant electrodes into the center of the brain that regulates eating behavior. A handful of obese patients had undergone lesions in a small area of the hypothalamus with some moderate success. Lozano was following the same target but applying high-frequency DBS to see if it would help curb the man's appetite. The patient had tried dieting and medicines but had refused the most modern dietary surgical intervention, gastric bypass.

In the operating room, Lozano's team stimulated the lead to make sure it reached its target. When the electrodes were stimulated on a specific lead, the fifty-year-old man said that he was experiencing a rather odd, déjà vu phenomenon, seeing himself around twenty years old and in a park with friends. The scene was in color, and he could make out the clothes that his friends were wearing. His girlfriend was there, and he was watching the scene rather than participanting. He could see that they were talking but couldn't make out their words. This specific autobiographical memory came under stimulation with three volts, 130 hertz, and sixty pulse widths. When the intensity of the electrical stimulation was ramped up to five volts, the scene became more vivid. But at this voltage he also experienced unpleasant warmth throughout his body, followed by sweat.

Lozano was intrigued by the memory. The man didn't know if it was something that actually had happened. But whenever this one lead was stimulated, the same experience came back. When the lead was turned off, the memory quickly evaporated.

To look more deeply into this odd effect, Lozano and his colleagues brought the patient back about two months later for a series of memory tests. He was shown 120 pairs of words on a computer screen and later asked to describe which pairs were more pleasant. Then he was asked whether he had seen the words in a pair or not. This same test was repeated a year after the initial surgery. During the test, the stimulator was turned either off or on. Lozano said that the patient was more likely to provide a "remember" response to a recognized pair of words when the stimulator was on—about 70 percent correct responses versus 43 percent when the stimulator was off.

The case got Lozano thinking about memory disorders and wondering if stimulation of certain areas of the hypothalamus could help in conditions like mild cognitive impairment, a precursor to Alzheimer's disease in many cases. With the finding of this surprising memory effect, Lozano said, "We have proof that we are driving the cognitive circuits." The team received approval from the hospital's investigational review board to operate on three patients with mild cognitive impairment, a condition marked by memory problems that fall somewhat short of normal in older people. The Canadian team also planned to write a study protocol to test deep brain stimulation in Alzheimer's patients.

The decision to investigate new conditions with deep brain stimulation has expanded well beyond what Irving Cooper could have imagined. In France, the father of high-frequency deep brain stimulation, Alim-Louis Benabid, also brought obese patients into surgery, and he began thinking about disorders of memory as well. He operated on his first severely depressed patient in 2008. In China, a team of specialists is using the technology to treat cocaine, opium, and morphine addiction. Italian surgeons have proposed using DBS to treat aggressive impulses.

Following the lead of Giovanni Broggi at the C. Besta National Neurological Institute in Milan, Italy, Kendall Lee, a neurosurgeon at the Mayo Clinic in Minnesota, used DBS to treat severe facial pain in almost a dozen patients beginning in 2006 and added cluster headaches to the list in 2008. He said that brain scans show the hypothalamus is hyperactive in patients with cluster headaches. Lee and his neurosurgical colleague Dudley Davis operated on three such patients by placing stimulating electrodes into the hypothalamus on one side of the brain. Lee reported that the procedure significantly reduced the frequency of these headaches. (European groups were also studying DBS for cluster headaches.)

The field may ultimately have to set guidelines and regulate the use of the technique. Lee operated on an eighteen-year-old man with Tourette syndrome, despite published recommendations that the experimental technique should not be carried out in patients under twenty-five. Tourette experts had said that DBS should be considered only if patients have reached adulthood with disabling symptoms that have not responded to available therapies. Normally, the tics begin in childhood but become less severe and, in many cases, disappear by the third decade of life. Lee said he had no idea that such recommendations had been published. The boy's parents had been involved in the decision to operate.

How far should DBS go? Are neurosurgeons justified in going after memory just because DBS repeatedly triggered a single snapshot of an experience that may or may not have happened? And one person's ability to remember pairs of words is no indication that invasive, risky DBS surgery will strengthen memory in people with mild cognitive impairment or Alzheimer's. As of 2009, using deep brain stimulation for anything other than movement disorders was still considered experimental. No one knows whether the technique will ultimately help people with obsessive-compulsive disorder or depression or cluster headaches or epilepsy. Studies are only beginning, and it will take years to find out whether the risks outweigh the benefits. "We have to be careful not to use a good tool unwisely," Benabid said. "It might have complications."

And as neuroscientists identify the circuits involved in other brain diseases—passing DBS leads in, around, and through the tissue of the exquisite human brain and identifying the effects of that procedure on the wide swath of cognitive activities and emotions—what systems will be put in place to ensure that these techniques are not used for pure human enhancement? It begins to seem that DBS may one day join a debate similar to that now raging over medications that can also boost mental performance in healthy people: should everyone have the option of strengthening healthy brain networks to feel or to think better than normal?

References

1 For a complete transcript of the Food and Drug Administration hearing, see http://www.fda.gov/ohrms/dockets/ac/97/transcpt/3273t1.pdf.

2 Stanley Finger, *Origins of Neuroscience: A History of Explorations into Brain Function* (New York: Oxford University Press, 2001), 225–226.

3 A more detailed description of these early events can be found in Jim Robbins, *A Symphony in the Brain: The Evolution of the New Brain Wave Biofeedback* (New York: Grove Press, 2001).

4 E. A. Spiegel, H. T. Wycis, M. Marks, and A. J. Lee, "Stereotaxic apparatus for operations on the human brain," *Science* 106 (1947): 349–350.

5 Michael L. J. Apuzzo, "New dimensions of neurosurgery in the realm of high technology: Possibilities, practicalities, realities," *Neurosurgery* 38(no. 4) (1996): 625–639.

6 E. Svennilson, A. Torvik, R. Lowe, and L. Leksell, "Treatment of Parkinsonism by stereotactic thermolesions in the pallidal region: A clinical evaluation of 81 cases," *Acta Psychiatrica Scandinavia* 35 (1960): 358–377.

7 P. L. Gildenberg, "The birth of stereotactic surgery: A personal retrospective;" *Neurosurgery* 54(no. 1) (2004): 199–207.

8 Kaushik Das, Deborah L. Benzil, Richard L. Rovit, Raj Murali, and William T. Couldwell, "Irving S. Cooper (1922–1985): A pioneer in functional neurosurgery," *Journal of Neurosurgery* 89 (1998): 865–873.

9 I. S. Cooper, *The Neurosurgical Alleviation of Parkinsonism* (Springfield Ill.: Charles S. Thomas, 1956).

10 Margaret Bourke-White, "Famous lady's indomitable fight," *Life,* June 22, 1959, 101–110.

11 "$1.8 million award for brain damage," *New York Times,* August 16, 1979, B2.

12 For more information on Irving S. Cooper, read *The Vital Probe: My Life as a Brain Surgeon* (New York: Norton, 1981. For more books and manuscripts by Cooper, see the reference section below.

13 Viartis, "History of Parkinson's disease," http://viartis.net/parkinsons.disease/history.htm.

14 J. William Langston et al., *Science* 225, no. 4669 (September 28, 1984): 1480–1482.

15 G. C. Davis, A. C. Williams, S. P. Markey, M. H. Ebert, E. D. Caine, C. M. Reichert, and I. J. Kopin, "Chronic parkinsonism secondary to intravenous injection of meperidine analogues," *Psychiatry Research* 1 (1979): 249–254.

16 The complete story of how MPTP was discovered is told by Langston and Jon Palfreman in *The Case of the Frozen Addicts* (New York: Pantheon, 1995).

17 M. B. Carpenter and A. Jayaraman, eds., *The Basal Ganglia II* (New York: Plenum, 1987): 415–427.

18 H. Bergman, T. Wichmann, and M. R. DeLong, "Reversal of experimental parkinsonism by lesions of the subthalamic nucleus," *Science* 249, no. 4975 (September 21, 1990): 1436–1438.

19 L. V. Laitinen, "My 50 years of interest in stereotactic and functional neurosurgery," *Stereotactic and Functional Neurosurgery* 77 (2001): 7–10.

20 R. L. Albin, A. B. Young, and J. B. Penney, "The functional anatomy of basal ganglia disorders," *Trends in Neuroscience* 12 (1989): 366–375.

21 J. L. Vitek, R. Bakay, A. Freeman, et al., "Randomized trial of pallidotomy versus medical therapy for Parkinson's disease," *Annals of Neurology* 53, no. 5 (2003): 558–569.

22 A. L. Benabid, P. Pollak, A. Louveau, S. Henry, and J. de Rougemont, "Combined (thalamotomy and stimulation) stereotactic surgery of the VIM thalamic nucleus for bilateral Parkinson's disease," *Applied Neurophysiology* 50 (1987): 344–346.

23 Satoshi Goto, Shuji Mita, and Yukitaka Ushio, "Bilateral pallidal stimulation for cervical dystonia: An optimal paradigm from our experiences," *Stereotactic and Functional Neurosurgery* 79 (2002): 221–227.

24 Jack El-Hai, *The Lobotomist* (Hoboken, N.J.: Wiley, 2005).

25 M. A. Jenike, L. Baer, T. Ballantine, et al., "Cingulotomy for refractory obsessive-compulsive disorder: A long-term follow-up of 33 patients," *Archives of General Psychiatry* 48 (1991): 548–555.

26 The World Health Organization's Global Burden of Disease Study published in *Global Burden of Disease and Risk Factor*, ed. Alan D. Lopez, Colin D. Mathers, Majid Ezzati, and Dean T. Jamison (Washington, D.C.: World Bank Publications, 2006)

27 B. P. Bejjani, P. Damier, et al., "Transient acute depression induced by high frequency deep-brain stimulation," *New England Journal of Medicine* 340 (1999): 1476–1480.

28 D. Malone, D. Dougherty, A. Rezai, et al., "Deep brain stimulation of the ventral capsule/ventral striatum for treatment-resistant depression," *Biological Psychiatry* (October 2008). [Online but not in print as yet. AU: volume number? page numbers?]

29 A. M. Lozano, H. S. Mayberg, et al., "Subcallosal Cingulate Gyrus Deep Brain Stimulation for Treatment-Resistant Depression," [My paper] *Biological Psychiatry* 64, no. 6 (2008): 461–467.

30 Yasin Temel and Veerle Visser-Vandewalle, "Surgery in Tourette syndrome," *Movement Disorders* 19, no. 1 (2004): 3–14.

31 Donald C. Shields, Ming L. Cheng, Alice W. Flaherty, John T. Gale, and Emad N. Eskandar, "Microelectrode-guided deep brain stimulation for Tourette syndrome: within-subject comparison of different stimulation Sites," *Stereotactic and Functional Neurosurgery* 86 (2008): 87–91.

32 Emily Stern, David A. Silbersweig, Kit-Yun Chee, Andrew Holmes, et al, "A functional neuroanatomy of tics in Tourette syndrome," *Archives of General Psychiatry* 57 (2000): 741–748.

33 To see a video of Jeffrey Matovic, go to: http://www.youtube.com/watch?v=y-iw_Xvh6G4.

34 Fran Simon, "Calming a storm in the brain," *Tulane University Magazine* March 9, 2006, http://www2.tulane.edu/ article_news_details.cfm?ArticleID=6319.

35 To learn more about Tourette's syndrome, visit the Tourette Syndrome Association's Web site at www.tsa-usa.org.

36 R. S. Fisher, S. Uematsu, G. L. Krauss, et al., "Placebo-controlled pilot study of centromedian thalamic stimulation in treatment of intractable seizures," *Epilepsia* 33 (1992): 841–851.

37 Ibid.

38 K. Vonck, P. Boon, E. Achten, J. De Reuck, and J. Caemaert, "Long-term amygdalohippocampal stimulation for refractory temporal lobe epilepsy," *Annals of Neurology* 52 (2002): 556–565.

39 H. U. Voss, A. M. Uluç, J. P. Dyke, et al., "Possible axonal regrowth in late recovery from the minimally conscious state," *Journal of Clinical Investigation* 116 no. 7 (2006): 2005–2011.

40 N. Schiff, "Behavioural improvements with thalamic stimulation after severe traumatic brain injury," *Nature* 448 (2007) 600–603.

41 M. S. Okun, N. P. Stover, et al., "Complications of gamma knife surgery for Parkinson disease," *Archives of Neurology* 58 (2001): 1995–2002.

Additional Resources
of Interest

Cooper, I. S. *It's Hard to Leave While the Music's Playing*. New York: Norton, 1977.

———. *The Vital Probe: My Life as a Brain Surgeon*. New York: Norton, 1981.

Cooper, Irving S., and associates. "St. Barnabas Symposium on surgical therapy of extrapyramidal disorders," *Journal of the American Geriatrics Society* (1956).

Cooper, Irving S. *The Neurological Alleviation of Parkinsonism*. Springfield, Ill.: Charles C. Thomas, 1956.

Hamani, Clement, et al. "Memory enhancement induced by hypothalamic/fornix deep brain stimulation. Brief communication," *Annals of Neurology*, 63, no. 1 (2008):119–123.

Merkel, R., et al. *Intervening in the Brain: Changing Psyche and Society, Ethics of Science and Technology Assessment*, Vol. 29. Berlin: Springer, 2007.

Okun, Michael S., et al. "Deep brain stimulation in the internal capsule and nucleus accumbens region: Responses observed during active and sham programming." *Journal of Neurology, Neurosurgery, and Psychiatry* 78 (2007):310–314.

Penfield, Wilder. *The Mystery of the Mind*. Princeton, N.J.: Princeton University Press, 1975.

Sacks, Oliver. *The Man Who Mistook His Wife for a Hat, and Other Clinical Tales*. New York: Summit Books, 1985.

Tarsay, Daniel, Jerrold Vitek, and Andres Lozano, eds. *Surgical Treatment of Parkinson's Disease and Other Movement Disorders*. Totowa, N.J.: Humana, 2003.

Twisted. DVD, directed by Laurel Chiten. Blind Dog Films, 2006.

Index

Other Dana Press Books
www.dana.org/news/danapressbooks

Books for General Readers

Brain and Mind

TRY TO REMEMBER: Psychiatry's Clash Over Meaning, Memory, and Mind
Paul R. McHugh, M.D.

Prominent psychiatrist and author Paul McHugh chronicles his battle to put right what has gone wrong in psychiatry. McHugh takes on such controversial subjects as "recovered memories," multiple personalities, and the overdiagnosis of PTSD.

Cloth • 300 pp • ISBN-13: 978-1-932594-39-3 • $25.00

CEREBRUM 2008: Emerging Ideas in Brain Science
Foreword by Carl Zimmer

The second annual anthology drawn from Cerebrum's highly regarded Web edition, Cerebrum 2008 brings together an international roster of scientists and other scholars to interpret the latest discoveries about the human brain and confront their implications.

Paper •225 pp • ISBN-13: 978-1-932594-33-1 • $14.95

CEREBRUM 2007: Emerging Ideas in Brain Science
Foreword by Bruce S. McEwen, Ph.D.

Paper • 243 pp • ISBN-13: 978-1-932594-24-9 • $14.95

Visit Cerebrum online at www.dana.org/news/cerebrum.

YOUR BRAIN ON CUBS: Inside the Heads of Players and Fans
Dan Gordon, Editor

Our brains light up with the rush that accompanies a come-from-behind win—and the crush of a disappointing loss. Brain research also offers new insight into how players become experts. Neuroscientists and science writers explore these topics and more in this intriguing look at talent and triumph on the field and our devotion in the stands.

6 illustrations.

Cloth • 150 pp • ISBN-13: 978-1-932594-28-7 • $19.95

THE NEUROSCIENCE OF FAIR PLAY:
Why We (Usually) Follow the Golden Rule
Donald W. Pfaff, Ph.D.

A distinguished neuroscientist presents a rock-solid hypothesis of why humans across time and geography have such similar notions of good and bad, right and wrong.

10 illustrations.

Cloth • 234 pp • ISBN-13: 978-1-932594-27-0 • $20.95

BEST OF THE BRAIN FROM SCIENTIFIC AMERICAN:
Mind, Matter, and Tomorrow's Brain

Floyd E. Bloom, M.D., Editor

Top neuroscientist Floyd E. Bloom has selected the most fascinating brain-related articles from *Scientific American* and *Scientific American Mind* since 1999 in this collection.
30 illustrations.

Cloth • 300 pp • ISBN-13: 978-1-932594-22-5 • $25.00

MIND WARS: Brain Research and National Defense

Jonathan D. Moreno, Ph.D.

A leading ethicist examines national security agencies' work on defense applications of brain science, and the ethical issues to consider.

Cloth • 210 pp • ISBN-10: 1-932594-16-7 • $23.95

THE DANA GUIDE TO BRAIN HEALTH:
A Practical Family Reference from Medical Experts (with CD-ROM)

Floyd E. Bloom, M.D., M. Flint Beal, M.D., and David J. Kupfer, M.D., Editors

Foreword by William Safire

A complete, authoritative, family-friendly guide to the brain's development, health, and disorders.
16 full-color pages and more than 200 black-and-white drawings.

Paper (with CD-ROM) • 733 pp • ISBN-10: 1-932594-10-8 • $25.00

THE CREATING BRAIN: The Neuroscience of Genius

Nancy C. Andreasen, M.D., Ph.D.

A noted psychiatrist and best-selling author explores how the brain achieves creative breakthroughs, including questions such as how creative people are different and the difference between genius and intelligence.
33 illustrations/photos.

Cloth • 197 pp • ISBN-10: 1-932594-07-8 • $23.95

THE ETHICAL BRAIN

Michael S. Gazzaniga, Ph.D.

Explores how the lessons of neuroscience help resolve today's ethical dilemmas, ranging from when life begins to free will and criminal responsibility.

Cloth • 201 pp • ISBN-10: 1-932594-01-9 • $25.00

A GOOD START IN LIFE:
Understanding Your Child's Brain and Behavior from Birth to Age 6

Norbert Herschkowitz, M.D., and Elinore Chapman Herschkowitz

The authors show how brain development shapes a child's personality and behavior, discussing appropriate rule-setting, the child's moral sense, temperament, language, playing, aggression, impulse control, and empathy.
13 illustrations.

Cloth • 283 pp • ISBN-10: 0-309-07639-0 • $22.95
Paper (Updated with new material) • 312 pp • ISBN-10: 0-9723830-5-0 • $13.95

BACK FROM THE BRINK:
How Crises Spur Doctors to New Discoveries about the Brain

Edward J. Sylvester

In two academic medical centers, Columbia's New York Presbyterian and Johns Hopkins Medical Institutions, a new breed of doctor, the neurointensivist, saves patients with life-threatening brain injuries.

16 illustrations/photos.

Cloth • 296 pp • ISBN-10: 0-9723830-4-2 • $25.00

THE BARD ON THE BRAIN:
Understanding the Mind Through the Art of Shakespeare and the Science of Brain Imaging

Paul M. Matthews, M.D., and Jeffrey McQuain, Ph.D. • *Foreword by Diane Ackerman*

Explores the beauty and mystery of the human mind and the workings of the brain, following the path the Bard pointed out in 35 of the most famous speeches from his plays.

100 illustrations.

Cloth • 248 pp • ISBN-10: 0-9723830-2-6 • $35.00

STRIKING BACK AT STROKE: A Doctor-Patient Journal

Cleo Hutton and Louis R. Caplan, M.D.

A personal account, with medical guidance from a leading neurologist, for anyone enduring the changes that a stroke can bring to a life, a family, and a sense of self.

15 illustrations.

Cloth • 240 pp • ISBN-10: 0-9723830-1-8 • $27.00

UNDERSTANDING DEPRESSION:
What We Know and What You Can Do About It

J. Raymond DePaulo, Jr., M.D., and Leslie Alan Horvitz

Foreword by Kay Redfield Jamison, Ph.D.

What depression is, who gets it and why, what happens in the brain, troubles that come with the illness, and the treatments that work.

Cloth • 304 pp • ISBN-10: 0-471-39552-8 • $24.95
Paper • 296 pp • ISBN-10: 0-471-43030-7 • $14.95

KEEP YOUR BRAIN YOUNG:
The Complete Guide to Physical and Emotional Health and Longevity

Guy M. McKhann, M.D., and Marilyn Albert, Ph.D.

Every aspect of aging and the brain: changes in memory, nutrition, mood, sleep, and sex, as well as the later problems in alcohol use, vision, hearing, movement, and balance.

Cloth • 304 pp • ISBN-10: 0-471-40792-5 • $24.95
Paper • 304 pp • ISBN-10: 0-471-43028-5 • $15.95

THE END OF STRESS AS WE KNOW IT

Bruce S. McEwen, Ph.D., with Elizabeth Norton Lasley • Foreword by Robert Sapolsky

How brain and body work under stress and how it is possible to avoid its debilitating effects.

Cloth • 239 pp • ISBN-10: 0-309-07640-4 • $27.95
Paper • 262 pp • ISBN-10: 0-309-09121-7 • $19.95

IN SEARCH OF THE LOST CORD:
Solving the Mystery of Spinal Cord Regeneration

Luba Vikhanski

The story of the scientists and science involved in the international scientific race to find ways to repair the damaged spinal cord and restore movement.

21 photos; 12 illustrations.

Cloth • 269 pp • ISBN-10: 0-309-07437-1 • $27.95

THE SECRET LIFE OF THE BRAIN

Richard Restak, M.D. • Foreword by David Grubin

Companion book to the PBS series of the same name, exploring recent discoveries about the brain from infancy through old age.

Cloth • 201 pp • ISBN-10: 0-309-07435-5 • $35.00

THE LONGEVITY STRATEGY:
How to Live to 100 Using the Brain-Body Connection

David Mahoney and Richard Restak, M.D. • Foreword by William Safire

Advice on the brain and aging well.

Cloth • 250 pp • ISBN-10: 0-471-24867-3 • $22.95
Paper • 272 pp • ISBN-10: 0-471-32794-8 • $14.95

STATES OF MIND: New Discoveries About How Our Brains Make Us Who We Are

Roberta Conlan, Editor

Adapted from the Dana/Smithsonian Associates lecture series by eight of the country's top brain scientists, including the 2000 Nobel laureate in medicine, Eric Kandel.

Cloth • 214 pp • ISBN-10: 0-471-29963-4 • $24.95
Paper • 224 pp • ISBN-10: 0-471-39973-6 • $18.95

The Dana Foundation Series on Neuroethics

DEFINING RIGHT AND WRONG IN BRAIN SCIENCE:
Essential Readings in Neuroethics

Walter Glannon, Ph.D., Editor

The fifth volume in The Dana Foundation Series on Neuroethics, this collection marks the five-year anniversary of the first meeting in the field of neuroethics, providing readers with the seminal writings on the past, present, and future ethical issues facing neuroscience and society.

Cloth • 350 pp • ISBN-10: 978-1-932594-25-6 • $15.95

HARD SCIENCE, HARD CHOICES:
Facts, Ethics, and Policies Guiding Brain Science Today

Sandra J. Ackerman, Editor

Top scholars and scientists discuss new and complex medical and social ethics brought about by advances in neuroscience. Based on an invitational meeting co-sponsored by the Library of Congress, the National Institutes of Health, the Columbia University Center for Bioethics, and the Dana Foundation.

Paper • 152 pp • ISBN-10: 1-932594-02-7 • $12.95

NEUROSCIENCE AND THE LAW: Brain, Mind, and the Scales of Justice

Brent Garland, Editor. With commissioned papers by Michael S. Gazzaniga, Ph.D., and Megan S. Steven; Laurence R. Tancredi, M.D., J.D.; Henry T. Greely, J.D.; and Stephen J. Morse, J.D., Ph.D.

How discoveries in neuroscience influence criminal and civil justice, based on an invitational meeting of 26 top neuroscientists, legal scholars, attorneys, and state and federal judges convened by the Dana Foundation and the American Association for the Advancement of Science.

Paper • 226 pp • ISBN-10: 1-032594-04-3 • $8.95

BEYOND THERAPY: Biotechnology and the Pursuit of Happiness
A Report of the President's Council on Bioethics

Special Foreword by Leon R. Kass, M.D., Chairman

Introduction by William Safire

Can biotechnology satisfy human desires for better children, superior performance, ageless bodies, and happy souls? This report says these possibilities present us with profound ethical challenges and choices. Includes dissenting commentary by scientist members of the Council.

Paper • 376 pp • ISBN-10: 1-932594-05-1 • $10.95

NEUROETHICS: Mapping the Field. Conference Proceedings

Steven J. Marcus, Editor

Proceedings of the landmark 2002 conference organized by Stanford University and the University of California, San Francisco, and sponsored by the Dana Foundation, at which more than 150 neuroscientists, bioethicists, psychiatrists and psychologists, philosophers, and professors of law and public policy debated the ethical implications of neuroscience research findings.
50 illustrations.

Paper • 367 pp • ISBN-10: 0-9723830-0-X • $10.95

Immunology

RESISTANCE: The Human Struggle Against Infection

Norbert Gualde, M.D., translated by Steven Rendall

Traces the histories of epidemics and the emergence or re-emergence of diseases, illustrating how new global strategies and research of the body's own weapons of immunity can work together to fight tomorrow's inevitable infectious outbreaks.

Cloth • 219 pp • ISBN-10: 1-932594-00-0 • $25.00

FATAL SEQUENCE: The Killer Within

Kevin J. Tracey, M.D.

An easily understood account of the spiral of sepsis, a sometimes fatal crisis that most often affects patients fighting off nonfatal illnesses or injury. Tracey puts the scientific and medical story of sepsis in the context of his battle to save a burned baby, a sensitive telling of cutting-edge science.

Cloth • 231 pp • ISBN-10: 1-932594-06-X • $23.95
Paper • 231 pp • ISBN-10: 1-932594-09-4 • $12.95

Arts Education

A WELL-TEMPERED MIND: Using Music to Help Children Listen and Learn

Peter Perret and Janet Fox • Foreword by Maya Angelou

Five musicians enter elementary school classrooms, helping children learn about music and contributing to both higher enthusiasm and improved academic performance. This charming story gives us a taste of things to come in one of the newest areas of brain research: the effect of music on the brain.

12 illustrations.

Cloth • 225 pp • ISBN-10: 1-932594-03-5 • $22.95
Paper • 225 pp • ISBN-10: 1-932594-08-6 • $12.00

Dana Press also offers several free periodicals dealing with brain science, arts education, and immunology. For more information, please visit www.dana.org.